The Greatest Diet on Earth

Nature's Lessons In Fulfilling Your Life's Desires

KAREN F. CURINGA

www.thegreatestdietonearth-karencuringa.com

Published by Globe Publishing
Salt Lake City, Utah

Globe Publishing
Salt Lake City, Utah DWS

ISBN #0-9726380-0-8

Cover: George Foster, Foster & Foster Inc.
Photographs: Drake Busath, Busath Photographers
Text: Clark Kidman, DTS
Editing: Lisa Workman

Printed in the United States by:
Alexander's
Lindon, Utah

About the Author

Karen Curinga is an author, speaker and consultant. Her book, The Greatest Diet On Earth, is based on the life transforming effects of consuming a predominantly raw plant-based food diet (a way of eating where one consumes mostly fresh fruits and fresh vegetables).

Karen has studied extensively, attended instructional workshops in the field of raw plant-based nutrition, as well as personally experienced, over the last eight years, the incredibly beneficial effects consuming a diet rich in raw plant-based foods has on the health and well-being of the body and the mind.

While maintaining this diet, she has eliminated severe allergies, arthritis, ulcers, bouts with depression and blood circulation problems from her life, while, at the same time, greatly enhancing clarity of mind. She has also experienced a medication-free, symptom-free menopause.

Karen realized the need for and was inspired to put her experience and knowledge into book form after continuous requests from individuals over the last eight years for her input and consultation regarding how they could make the change to a raw plant-based food diet and experience the life transforming effects of weight loss and maintenance, health and incredible energy that were so evident in her life. She currently provides private consultations.

Karen is also a contributing writer for several health publications and promotes and speaks to groups on the benefits of a raw plant-based lifestyle. She is a member of the Advisory Board of a College Advisory Council, a Business Consultant and a licensed, certified Mediator. She is also currently working on her next, "soon to be released" book. Although she was raised in California, she now resides in Salt Lake City, Utah.

Special Acknowledgements

No accomplishment in life is ever a one-person process. I want to thank every person that contributed so graciously to the development of this book and supported me along the way.

A special thanks to Kellie who lovingly pushed, encouraged and supported me every inch of the way. Special thanks also to Mitch, Rudy, Bob and Kelly who provided continual belief and support in me and in this project.

A special thanks to Kathleen who provided constant support, assistance, information and friendship.

I would also like to thank George, Drake, Lisa, Clark, Barry and J'nel for their assistance, professionalism, friendship and sense of humor on this journey.

Table of Contents

PREFACE

Welcome to *The Greatest Diet On Earth*. By opening the pages of this book you have taken the first step into the new world that is awaiting you. Just as a diet is actually an ongoing way of living, not a temporary fix, life is a continual process of growth. Each of us is here to consistently unfold and develop to the best of our abilities. It is not only an opportunity we are given. It is our responsibility to life. Being the best we can be does not mean pitting each of us in a competitive battle to declare a winner. It means that each one of us becomes truly beautiful when we discover our own unique stride. We each contribute a special thread to the tapestry of life and are an essential part in our own way since we are all woven together and interconnected.

As we follow the principles contained in the following pages of this book, a true awakening begins to take place within us. As we start to observe and feel the wonderful physical changes happening to our body, we also become aware of the mental clarity and power that replaces the confusion and doubt that previously existed. We find that as we take care of our body in the way it was intended, many of the conditions and ailments we have accepted as normal all our lives do not even have to occur. It becomes clear that we are not helpless victims in a world beyond our control. We transition easily and calmly into the knowledge of how powerful we each are and we begin to see that we have great control in what we allow to enter our life. Life is a series of choices and we now are able to confidently make the choices that are in our best interest. We find that this is not an act of selfishness, but an act of inspiration to others that encourages them to do and be their best. We are each meant to shine.

Let's begin.

INTRODUCTION

How This Program Developed

*"Vitality and beauty are gifts of Nature for those
who live according to its laws."*
— Leonardo Da Vinci

This is the beginning of the last food program you will ever
need and the start of a way of living that will amaze you more
and more the longer it remains a part of your life. Before we get
started, take a moment to answer the following questions.
In the last several years:

- Has your clothing size dropped several sizes? Have you
  maintained that ideal size without fluctuation?
- Have you experienced menopause without medication
  and yet haven't suffered from a SINGLE uncomfortable
  symptom such as sweats, irritability, etc.?
- Has your energy and stamina risen to the level of two "normal" people?
- Have allergies that you suffered with for years disappeared?
- Has arthritis in your hands and legs disappeared?
- Have persistent circulation problems in your hands and
  feet completely disappeared?
- Have you stopped experiencing any type of headaches or
  sinus problems?
- Have you risen to a new level of self-respect and self-esteem?
- Do you have a clarity of thinking that you had not previ-
  ously experienced?
- Has your spiritual consciousness expanded to a degree
  you did not think possible?

- Have you been able to eat as much as you want without gaining weight?
- Has your grocery bill actually gone down?
- Have you stopped taking medication of any kind, including aspirin?
- Have you found you can get by easily on less sleep per night?
- Have you found more fulfillment and joy in your daily experiences?
- Have fine lines on your skin disappeared and your skin completely cleared?
- Has your hair thickened and the nails you had completely given up on grown?
- Have acquaintances and strangers stopped you and asked what your secret is for maintaining a thin body?
- Have others asked you to explain to them how you eat to maintain such a high energy level?
- Have your medical exams returned from the labs with a literal "thumbs up" on them?
- Have you found a peace within yourself and a belief in yourself that you have been waiting for all your life?

You might be saying to yourself, "Those things don't happen to anyone as they age." I'm here to tell you that *every one* of the above experiences has happened to me. As of this very day your life can begin improving in extraordinary ways. In the last eight years I have followed a raw plant-based food lifestyle and have experienced — and continue to experience — all of the above wonderful changes in my life and even more. It is the combination of not only what I eat, but also the amounts of food eaten that have changed my life. To my joy and excitement, I have personally discovered that we each have an unlimited ability to direct and control the outcome of our life... physically, psychologically and spiritually.

Eight years ago, I was not even sure that I wanted to go on living. It took all my strength to get out of bed in the morning and pull back the curtains. I was going through a divorce. My mother was in the last stages of breast cancer. My weight was increasing by the minute. The financial security and comfortable lifestyle I had become accustomed to had vanished. I had no purpose. I felt helpless, continually fatigued and panicked about my future. I felt unattractive and ill prepared to face what might lie ahead. *And then my life changed.*

They say the darkest hour is just before dawn... and that was so in my case. I am still not exactly sure what happened. No visions appeared, no great epiphanies. I only know that one day I woke up and felt I was in such a hole, I had to start digging my way out. After all, I had two children. I wanted to be an example to them... not a burden.

At that time I believed that the majority of things happening around me were not within my control (a belief which has been drastically altered) so I decided to start with the one thing I believed was within my immediate control... my eating habits and my health. I believe I must have had some type of a spiritual awakening because for the first time in my life, I was not trying to give up bad habits... the bad habits were giving me up... almost effortlessly.

Through the years up to that point I had endured my share of battles with weight. I had done the yo-yo dieting thing over and over again. I had searched unendingly for that one way of eating that I could stick with and would provide me with beauty and sleekness. In the early days I didn't even care about the health aspect...just as long as it would keep me thin. But I could never find that "perfect" diet or way of eating. And I also noticed that no one I knew ever seemed to find the "perfect" diet either. At one point my health became a serious concern when my menstrual cycles stopped for no reason (I was not pregnant) and had to be put on birth control pills (hormones) to try to regulate my cycle. It was later determined that strenuous dieting had been the cause.

When I initially started making changes in my life, I admit that my motives were vanity driven. My greatest concern was in losing the excess weight I had gained. I was looking for work and wanted to look my best. I also needed more energy and wanted to feel better about myself as a person. If someone would have told me at the time I began this program what the results would be, I would probably have dismissed them as some "food fanatic." At the risk of receiving this label myself, I had to share this information with as many as would listen. Every single area of my life has been changed so dramatically for the better, that I feel like life is just beginning.

In the past few years have you watched, seemingly helpless, diet after diet, as your clothing size continued to increase? Have you just accepted that this is your destiny as you age? It doesn't have to be that way.

Within six months of following a living food way of eating, I had dropped several sizes. My clothing size has now stabilized at a size that is ideal for me. What cannot be emphasized enough here is that it has not fluctuated in eight years. On this program, each person reaches his or her own individual ideal weight and size as it relates to their bone structure and height. As the introductory questions indicated, I also eat as much as I want without gaining weight. I have the energy of two people. My hair and fingernails grow healthy and strong. I have gone through menopause with absolutely no symptoms (i.e., hot flashes, sweats, irritability, etc.) *and* no medications. I no longer experience the symptoms of arthritis. I feel better now than I did when I was 21. I don't "do" aerobics or any strenuous exercise, just moderate amounts of exercise. My medical check-ups have come back with exclamation marks on them and comments such as, "Whatever you are doing... keep doing it!" I take *no* medication whatsoever... not even aspirin. The severe allergies I previously had forced me to sleep in a sitting position and caused sinus headaches. Now I am free of the debilitating allergy symptoms that affected my breathing, sleeping and energy level.

I may be slim now, but believe me, I have been where you are. I say that because I don't believe you would be reading this book if you were not at a point in your life where you are ready for some major changes.

I was inspired to write this book for several reasons:

1. The information in this book changed my life, my self-esteem and brought me joy in ways that I cannot adequately convey in words... and I am *passionate* about it.

2. During the years I have followed this program, people

have continually asked me to tell them how I consistently keep my weight down and my energy up.

3. I have lived this program for eight years now without fluctuation. I know beyond any doubt that it works and brings magical results, not only in weight maintenance, but in clarity of mind and spirit. I have also become acquainted with a calm power within me that was an unanticipated bonus.

4. Because I am just like you. If my life can change like it has, then so can yours. I was the "Queen of Lack of Self-Discipline." This new way of living feeds not only your body, but your soul. It is the lifestyle Nature intended. There are no mathematical calculations, no special, expensive foods you need to buy which you will need to wean yourself off from if you ever go back to "normal" eating, no expensive customized diet that needs to be developed or formulated specifically for you. This plan works for everyone: man, woman and child.

We are rapidly moving to an exciting point in our existence where we understand the great importance of the mind/body connection. Scientists and physicists have shown and continue to show us that *we are what we think*. We are also entering into an era where we can realize that we are what we *eat* as well. As the thought of living to a ripe old age becomes a reality, we can choose to live it in health, joy, activity and beauty where we are in control of our lives, or we can hope that the medical community will be able to provide us with enough medications and chemicals (to preserve us). At that point, we are not in control of our own life — the medical community is.

We are also looking at the cost of prevention vs. the cost of cure. Will you be able to afford the high price you will pay, not only in terms of health, but in medical costs for trying to cure what could more than likely have been avoided in the first place? You've heard the saying that the definition of insanity is doing the same thing over and over but expecting a different result. If you truly want a better life and better health for yourself, you will need to make the necessary changes.

The choice is ultimately yours.

There are many in the world today who would say that man has fallen from grace, that we as a race could not get much lower. I would disagree. I am not a Pollyanna, but I feel that the tremendous strides we are making in technology and science are indications that we, as a race, are ready to make another great leap intellectually. Reflective of that new awakening of intelligence is the fact that we are now realizing the wonderful powers and abilities inherent in each of us to create the life that we desire. We cannot control everything around us, but we can greatly change our immediate environment and ourselves by monitoring our thought processes. What all the great religious teachings (including the Bible) have been telling us all along, science and physics is now proving beyond any reasonable doubt. Our thought processes, both individually and collectively, create our world. Being alive at this point of time and space is a true gift. We are experiencing a reality that appeared impossible to earlier generations.

Startling new statistics reported in the October 9, 2002 issue of *USA Today* revealed that 64.5% of American adults are overweight or obese, according to *The National Health and Nutrition Examination Survey.* This survey is considered to be the most definitive assessment of American's weight due to the length and size of the study and because people's height and weight are actually measured. In the article Cynthia Ogden, an epidemiologist with the National Center for Health Statistics and an author of published studies in the *Journal of the American Medical Association,* states, "We want to emphasize that the problem of obesity and (being) overweight for adults and kids is getting worse." Samuel Klein, President of the North American Association for the Study of Obesity states in the article, "The medical costs of treating obesity-related disease will cause a considerable strain on the health care system and the economy."

Obesity is a problem of epidemic proportions in America. This ironically exists in a country obsessed with dieting, strenuous exercise and every kind of fat-free food known to man. In a study done by Susan B. Roberts, Ph.D., Chief of the Energy Metabolism Laboratory at Tufts University in Massachusetts, showed that in 1973 about 100 new processed baked products were introduced in the United States. Twenty years later, that number had grown to 1,500 new products. Too much choice may be one factor in the prevalence of obesity. "If I give you three different kinds of cookies, you'll eat more than if I give you one kind," says Roberts. She goes on to state that "portion sizes in America are geared to lumberjacks... it's easy to overeat. The average person may also be unaware that low-fat foods are often extremely high in calories."

Spending on health care in America has risen:
from .... $47 billion in 1960
to .... $360 billion in 1984
to .... $883 billion in 1993

Corporations are spending more on health care for their employees which is then passed on to the consumer by the increased cost of products. According to a United Nations world survey of health, out of 79 countries surveyed, the health of the people of the United States rated at the very bottom.

As mentioned earlier, technology is moving at lightning speed and we are experiencing advancements heretofore unknown to man. We can take a tuck here, a nip there and ingest mounds of medication to lose weight. The fact still remains that Americans are getting more obese, including our children.

I happened to be shopping in a large, rather exclusive, nationally known department store a few months ago and could not find any business suits in my size. When I questioned the salesperson, she told me that the buyer for the store had decided to discontinue the purchase of that size clothing because there were so few people who could wear them any longer. Instead, the buyer had decided to increase the quantity of larger sizes because the average woman purchaser for their store has become increasingly heavier. So much for the success of all our fat-free foods and fad diets.

I am not here to convince you of anything. That is something you must do for yourself. I know this way of living has changed every aspect of my life and thinking. When I began my journey, I spent countless hours diligently researching information that became the foundation of this lifestyle change. My hope is to provide you with enough information that you will be inspired to attempt this journey for yourself. It is a journey well worth taking.

The Laws of Nature are simple and straightforward. When you acknowledge and accept them, they become an ally, not an enemy. You can throw away your scales and calorie counters. Nature has already made the calculations for you. Nature has provided us with foods that are easy to prepare, colorful to the eye, and relatively inexpensive when compared to the processed or "fast" foods that make up the majority of the standard American diet. By the way, the standard American diet has been referred to as SAD. Hmm. Do you think this is a coincidence?

PART 1

Why This Diet Is *The Greatest Diet on Earth*

CHANGING YOUR LIFE, NOT YOUR "DIET"

"Nothing will benefit human health and increase the chances for survival of life on earth as much as the evolution to a vegetarian diet."
— Albert Einstein

I am going to go out on a limb here and make the assumption that you have had at least one diet failure. That is, you have, in good faith, previously attempted some widely publicized *diet system*. You may have even successfully reached the personal weight that you had set as your goal. But then it happened. That *diet system* was completed, you went back to your "real world" old way of eating. The pounds started creeping back and - voila! There you were again. Back to where you started. More than a little depressed, feeling like a failure, your self-esteem dinged once again. You kick yourself for not maintaining the weight loss, not realizing that the whole thing was just a "temporary fix." The reality is that you couldn't have maintained that diet system forever, so you were doomed to failure once you went back to the old way of living that had created the problem in the first place! I can appreciate this because I have been there too.

The Greatest Diet on Earth reflects the true meaning of the word 'diet' from the Greek word 'diaeta' — a way of life. When we have a clear understanding of what a diet truly is, we then can logically see that fad food weight loss programs are not true diets. The Greatest Diet on Earth is the answer you are seeking and this is why:

1. This way of eating is not a temporary fix. It allows you to eat the normal, God-given food we were meant to consume and it will become a wonderful way of life. You don't quit this lifestyle when you reach your ideal weight. This way of eating is a way of life where you are always the one making the choices and you are always in control.

2. Most diets are based on cutting down on calories or exercising rigorously, which can be especially tough for those getting older or in fragile physical condition. But I can tell you after years of maintaining my ideal weight and re-

ceiving wonderful check-up results, you can throw away the calorie counters and scales. Scales can be instant-depressants. With this way of eating, your body will lose the appropriate fat but will receive all the necessary nutrients — plus you will be hydrating your system and slowing the aging process. You can maintain moderate, enjoyable types of exercise such as walking. Your clothing will continue to grow looser as you move to your ideal weight and the increasing energy level will be enough indication that you are successfully shedding the unwanted pounds.

3. Calorie counters are completely unnecessary because Nature has already done all the calculating when you eat a raw-plant-based diet. It is very easy to follow this plan.

4. You will not experience hunger because you are never deprived with this way of eating. Eat until you are perfectly satisfied. You will only get *healthier*, not *heavier*.

5. Statistics have shown us that fad diets just don't work. It is said that less than five percent of those who initially lose weight actually keep it off. These types of results are stressful mentally and are very stressful to your body. Diet pills are absolutely no answer. Their potential harm to the body far outweighs any short-term weight loss.

6. Statistics are beginning to come in showing that with each new generation brought up on junk and processed foods, the mental and physical ailments tend to multiply. This is no coincidence. We, as parents, love our children and one of our foremost desires is to help prepare them for life. What better way than to instill sound minds and bodies? Since many of our "heroes" hype junk and processed foods on TV and Madison Avenue's approach to marketing does not appear to be changing anytime soon, it is up to us, as parents, to guide those receptive, impressionable and eager young minds in the direction that will serve them best.

7. This plant-based diet involves no medication of any kind. In fact, I found that the longer I followed this way of eating, the less medication I needed. Today I take no medications whatsoever. I don't even take aspirin. It is not necessary.

8. The idea underlying this entire way of eating is *KEEP IT SIMPLE*. What a refreshing idea!

Maybe the most important way this plan for life differs from the standard fad diets out there is that this offers a true way to change your life. You will definitely lose the weight and it is a wonderful feeling of accomplishment. However, this weight loss may even become secondary to the wonderful discovery of mental clarity. It's not about the pounds. That ends up merely being a very pleasant by-product.

As you rise to a higher level of living that allows you to truly see and feel your self-worth, you will find yourself making better decisions in your life, being more connected to the world around you and wanting to take more calculated risks toward fulfilling your goals and dreams that you previously lacked the confidence to take.

LOSE THE SCALES, LOSE THE CALCULATOR – GET WHAT YOUR BODY NEEDS FROM NATURE

The February 9, 2001 issue of *Living and Raw Foods* magazine reported:

> "After the most extensive study on nutrition ever undertaken by the government, the U.S. Senate Select Committee on Nutrition and Human Needs concluded in its 1978 report entitled "Diet and Killer Diseases," that the average American diet is responsible for the development of chronic degenerative diseases such as heart disease, arteriosclerosis, cancer, diabetes, stroke, etc."

That was in 1978. While our medical treatment has improved since that time, processed foods have increased at an alarming rate in both the number of products available and in the amount consumed by Americans.

Each cell in your body is a living, highly organized, thinking organism. You cannot fool the cells of your body. What you put into your body either meets the needs of those cells or it doesn't. There are no trick questions. You can't feed your body toxins and expect it to make nutrients out of nothing. This isn't a magic show and your cells are not magicians. They also live by Nature's Laws. If you put bad in, you get bad out. If you put good in, you get good out. It's that simple. Yet intelligent men and women continually pump toxic, carcinogenic, dead substances into their bodies and expect the cells of their body to create magic. They blame their body for turning on them when their health disintegrates or diseases appear. If I gave you two cotton swabs and a string of dental floss and asked you to convert it into a Porsche, you just couldn't do it. No matter how well organized or dedicated you were. (Well, maybe McGuyver could… but seriously). You can't expect your cells to provide you with glowing skin, shiny hair, strong nails, a healthy body and endless energy when you give it dead building blocks with which to work.

There came a point where it dawned on me that the natural way to health and fitness was the *simple* way. There are many people who make the idea and process of attaining a desired weight and level of health much more complicated than it actually is. In order to participate in their program you have so many rules and restrictions that you are lost in a maze before you begin. I believe most diet programs put their focus on the wrong things, the numbers of calories, pounds, etc. What we should be focusing on is the true joy that comes from feeling well and being full of energy and focusing on what foods work together in our bodies and what foods don't. When we finally realize that Nature gave each of us the intelligence and ability to discern what is good for us by listening to our bodies we will find a wonderful power and sense of control over our own lives that fills us with a feeling of freedom. Freedom from being controlled by external factors. Freedom to be who we are meant to be. Freedom to feel the enjoyment of life that Nature meant as a normal state of being.

When we finally wake up to the fact that we cannot fool the laws of Nature and accept that we are worthy of treating ourselves well, our world literally turns around. Your body is a part of you. It is not a thing that you either treat well or poorly. It is literally *you*. Treat it kindly and with respect and it will reward you in a multitude of ways.

Before explaining my personal view of this food program, I

am fully aware that most of us live busy lives with time concerns and possibly a family to cook for. Most of us do not have the luxury of spending our days lounging on the beach or by the pool, having our meals prepared and served to us as per our specifications.

We need to simplify our lives. It is unfortunate, however, that the media has bombarded us with messages that lead us to believe that the way to simplify our lives is to cram ourselves full of "ready to eat" processed foods. Americans are becoming more obese each year. But the real heavyweights are the diet and processed food industries. Processed foods are but one more example of man's assumption that he can do a better job than Nature. In the process, we make things far more complicated than they need to be. In our assumptions we make errors that will take generations to correct if, in fact, it is possible to correct them at all.

Our foods are pumped full of chemicals. They are deep fried in grease that has been reheated over and over again (which not only clogs your arteries, but is full of carcinogens). They are void of any water content, full of salt (dehydrating) or sugar (toxic), and mucus forming. What does it say when the food that makes up the majority of the average American's diet can live on a shelf for 5 years and not even attract the interest of an insect? Doesn't that shake you up just a little? The final nail in the coffin, so to speak, is that we will pay a premium price not only in terms of dollars, but also in terms of health.

The truth is that we are not really saving time or money. By pumping toxic substances into our systems, the preparation time we save by purchasing fast foods today will surely be equivalent to or exceed the time lost on the other end of our lives. The dollar cost of processed foods can only be multiplied many times by the future health care costs which will come about from lack of nutrition being supplied to our systems. The potential cost of not taking care of ourselves is staggering. We now see generations growing up that don't even know a life without some type of processed food at every meal. Take a look around you. How many children do you see eating an apple, banana or an orange for a snack? Most children don't even think in terms of choosing fresh fruit for a snack. It is more than a little disconcerting.

My work and lifestyle often puts me in situations where I am also faced with the "rubber chicken" lunches and receptions. I attend social gatherings where eating a healthy meal is not a major concern. What I do in these situations is simple. I still try to fill 90-95% of my plate with the foods I normally eat and allow 5-10% for the other foods that I normally do not eat. And while I am not a fanatic, I truly am passionate about this way of eating because I *know* beyond any doubt after living both lifestyles that the program of eating I follow today provides me with a weight, energy and health level that I only dreamed of in the past.

The true pleasure that comes from feeling so good, remaining at a stable weight with no extra fat on your body, and maintaining an extremely high energy level is something that cannot be explained in mere words. It must be experienced to be truly appreciated. It is never too late to start. Your body and your mind will respond in ways you can't imagine.

My personal food program has been developed over the past eight years through voluminous amounts of study, experiments in food types and combinations and how my body felt and reacted when consuming them. I have found over the years that the best plan for me is to follow a diet of approximately 95-100% raw foods. My diet consists mostly of raw fruits and vegetables and juices made from them. I also include a limited amount of soy and grain products. The soy in my diet is mostly tofu, but many soy products are available and will be discussed later in the book. Any grain products in my diet are in the form of sprouted grains. Once the grain has sprouted, it is easier to digest. I have eliminated dairy products and meat from my diet. I drink 3-4 quarts of pure, filtered water each day. I include both organic flax seed and olive oils each day to cover my Omega 3, 6 and 9 needs. I don't take any supplements because I feel that it is more effective to get all my vitamins and minerals through live foods. On rare occasions I include cold-water fish (mostly salmon). Meat, dairy products and grains are all acidic and mucus producing in the body. This mucus clogs organs just as cholesterol clogs arteries and veins.

When I first started following this program, I didn't know where it would lead. I only knew that I had to make a lifestyle change. No one I knew lived this philosophy or lifestyle. There was no one to confer with so I just kept searching and researching on my own. I voraciously studied everything I could get my hands on that had anything to do with health improvement. I attended lectures, seminars and workshops. The more I read and experimented, the more I knew that this way of eating was the right and natural way to care for our bodies. I think most of the people I knew thought that I had gone off the deep end. A lot of good spirited ribbing was done at my expense. But after a while, these same people started asking me what I was doing and how I was eating. They wanted to know why I had so much energy at the end of the day when they were worn out. They also wanted to know why I was successful at keeping weight off while they were struggling unsuccessfully to maintain. Their clothing size kept growing larger while mine stayed constant. These questions were also fielded by young women in their early 20's and by men as well. They could see that something good was working for me and wanted to know what it was and how it worked.

MANAGING MENOPAUSE

According to statistics, approximately 50 percent of women experience the onset of menopause between their mid-forties and fifty. This marks the beginning of the end of menstruation and a woman's reproductive years. Due to a record number of baby boomers now reaching mid-life, it has been estimated that by the year 2015, approximately 50 percent of U.S. women may be menopausal. This means that many women may spend up to a third or more of their lives beyond the age of menopause. With all the controversy that surrounds Hormone Replacement Therapy (HRT), it is a valid question to ask whether women are willing to spend that time on medication that may alleviate menopausal symptoms, but put their lives at risk in other areas, such as heart disease and cancer.

Women are now seeking a natural, healthy way to address these symptoms. They want to assume more control over their lives and the decisions as to how they will live them. The more informed we are, the better choices we can make for ourselves.

We, as Americans, are now realizing that moving into menopause does not have to be a depressing sign of aging. Older women of other cultures are honored and their maturity and wisdom is acknowledged, as is their beauty. The world today is full of absolutely beautiful, confident, successful women who are over 50 years of age. Life is full of continual change. Embrace life for the positive opportunities it provides. Most of us have spent the majority of our life, up to this point, taking care of others. This is the time to take care of ourselves. A time for rediscovering who we are, what our purpose is, what we want to accomplish, and developing our hidden talents. This is a time to take charge not only of our bodies, but of our lives.

The medical community tells us that there is a slowing of metabolism and a decline in estrogen levels during menopause that can contribute to weight gain and weight re-distribution. While this is a common symptom of menopause, the good news is that it is not written in stone. I am proof of that. I have traveled the menopause journey and have not experienced any weight gain or re-distribution of body weight. I attribute this entirely to the types of food I have consumed. It was the only thing I radically changed during my menopausal years.

When I first started putting together my own raw-plant-based diet, I started including tofu. I liked the flavor and knew that it was an alternative to the meat and dairy I had been eating.

As I had mentioned earlier, I have been eating my particular plant-based diet for about eight years. About four years ago I began the transition through menopause. What makes my experience unique is that while my friends were experiencing agonizing symptoms, I was experiencing no ill effect or discomfort. At the time, my physician could not believe that I could possibly go through menopause without the weight gain, hot flashes, headaches, night sweats, mood swings, tender breasts, etc., that are all common physical complaints of menopausal women. I must admit I was a bit perplexed as to why my menopausal experience was so different from anyone I knew. At that time, I knew no one who ate like I did. All I knew was that I felt great and the tests from my check-ups corroborated that. In addition to eating raw plant-based foods, soy, and increasing water consumption in my diet, I had given up sugar, salt, caffeine, alcohol, processed foods and fats (that were not of plant origin). To this day, I still experience no postmenopausal symptoms. I feel I am living proof that the way we eat can make a stunning difference in how we experience this inevitable change in our life.

There are those who ask me whether they should be concerned about eating soy products after seeing articles questioning soy products and their effects on estrogen levels in the body. In the May-June 2000 issue of *FDA Consumer* magazine, John Henkel of the FDA reports, "Much of the research to date has examined dietary soy in the form of *whole* foods such as tofu, "soymilk", or as soy protein added to foods, and the public health community mostly concurs that these whole foods can be worthwhile additions to a healthy diet. The recently raised concerns, however, focus on *specific components* of soy, such as the soy isoflavones daidzein and genistein, *not the whole food or intact soy protein*. These chemicals, available over the counter in pills and powders, are often advertised as dietary supplements for use by women to help lessen menopausal symptoms such as hot flashes."

In the same issue of *FDA Consumer*, Margo Woods, D.Sc., Associate Professor of Medicine at Tufts University, says her concerns are centered mainly on isoflavone *supplements* and that she's "much more comfortable" recommending soy as a whole food. She says, "There are probably hundreds of protective compounds in soy (foods). It's just too big a leap to assume a pill could do the same thing." Ms. Woods has studied soy's effects in postmenopausal women. Isoflavones generally tend to balance estrogen levels.

In the October 22, 2002 issue of *About Nutrition*, an interview was conducted with Dr. Mark Messina, Ph.D., a well-respected soy researcher and author. Dr. Messina states, "There is a legitimate concern about whether soy is contraindicated for women with ER+ breast cancer. Recently I have concluded that it is unlikely that soy is a problem for these women. My view, among other things, is based on the relationship between estrogen and breast cancer risk and a recent study that found that soy did not increase breast cell proliferation in premenopausal women as was initially reported."

Kenneth Setchell, a pediatrics professor at Children's Hospital in Cincinnati was reported in the October issue of abcnews.com as saying, "There have been literally hundreds of thousand of infants that have been raised on those soy formulas. Some of those infants would be well into their late 30's, early 40's now. And you know, I don't see evidence of tremendous numbers of cases where there are abnormalities."

As with anything in life, moderation is the key. For example, I have consumed only 2-3 ounces of tofu per day for years, yet I have still received the benefits of soy.

Studies also show that foods rich in boron appear to boost estrogen levels in postmenopausal women. Apples, pears, grapes, peaches, raisins, dates, soybeans, almonds, hazelnuts, and honey are rich in boron.

Cut out coffee and cigarettes. They deplete the body of estrogen. Caffeine consumption has also been linked to hot flashes. It also is a diuretic and contributes to fluid loss in the body.

Interesting Fact

An interesting but rather disturbing fact is that foreign estrogens called xenoestrogens are leached into our foods from plastic bags and pesticides.

What should you eat?
- Soy products (tofu, soymilk, tempeh, soy cheese). Tofu contains no cholesterol, no saturated fat, and is high in naturally occurring antioxidants.
- Ground flax seeds or flax seed oil (good source of phytoestrogens and Omega 3 fatty acids).
- Lots of dark green leafy vegetables (romaine lettuce, spinach, kale - also good sources of calcium).
- Cold water fish such as salmon, tuna, sardines, halibut.
- Eat several small meals per day.
- Drink plenty of water.

What should you avoid?
- Refined white sugar products.
- Salt. Be sure to check labels and avoid adding salt to foods. Fruits, vegetables and grains contain all the natural salt you will ever need.
- Processed Foods.
- Saturated Fats.
- Caffeine. Increases loss of calcium, can trigger hot flashes, can cause rise in blood pressure, encourages pancreas to release more insulin causing the blood sugar to drop making you feel hungry and increasing the odds of a food binge.
- Alcohol. Interferes with mineral absorption, can trigger hot flashes, depletes the body of vitamins A, B and C, can lead to premature wrinkling of the skin.
- Cigarettes. Increases risk of osteoporosis, speeds up the aging of the skin.
- Red meat.
- All other high stress foods: white flour products, sugar, black pepper, monosodium glutamate (MSG), and very hot spices (they may actually worsen hot flashes).

Always avoid negative thinking. Take control of your thoughts, stay optimistic and realize your own self-worth.

FOODS AND MENOPAUSAL SYMPTOMS	
Symptom	Foods
Hot Flashes	Trigger foods: Salt, sugar, spicy/hot foods, coffee, chocolate, tea, cola drinks, alcohol (These should be avoided for *all* symptoms.) Include: Soy-based products & citrus fruits.
Night Sweats	Avoid same as above. Eat a very light evening meal.

Vaginal and Urinary Symptoms	Keep bladder flushed by drinking at least 2-3 quarts of pure water each day. Cranberry juice may also help.
Muscle & Joint Pain and Stiffness	Consume more calcium through soy based foods, fish and dark greens.
Skin (dry/wrinkles)	Drink 3 quarts of water each day. Eat plenty of fresh vegetables and fruits to get enough Vitamin A, B, C and E. Take 2 tablespoons cold pressed flax seed oil per day.
Stomach Bloating and Bowel Symptoms	Drink 3 quarts of pure water each day. Eat plenty of fiber rich foods such as dark-green leafy vegetables, legumes, brown rice, and whole grain pasta.
Breast Discomfort	Appears to correlate with low levels of essential fatty acids and high consumption of saturated fats. Eat avocados, take flax seed oil, olive oil. Evening Primrose oil has been recorded to be effective is reducing breast pain.
Emotional Symptoms	Avoid trigger foods listed above, drink plenty of pure water, exercise.

The Success of Soy

Hormone Replacement Therapy (HRT) is a very controversial subject at this time. The known long-term benefits of HRT are increases in protection against heart disease and osteoporosis. However, the lining of the uterus can build up, thus increasing your chances of getting endometrial cancer or cancer of the uterus if estrogen is taken alone. To protect against this, progesterone (which keeps the uterine lining from building up) is also given. However, progesterone can somewhat decrease the health benefits of estrogen. These treatments may have side effects of their own such as bloating, nausea, mood changes, breast tenderness and headaches, which may be worse than the menopausal symptoms.

Common symptoms of menopause are hot flashes, night sweats, vaginal dryness, and weight gain.

When I decided to change my life, I had read a little about soy products but knew very little about them. Actually, I had never even eaten tofu or tempeh. They were "exotic foods" and I had no idea how to prepare them.

Today, although I consume only a small amount, soy products (mainly tofu) are a essential part of my diet. I feel strongly that soy has played a large role in my lack of menopausal and postmenopausal symptoms.

About four years ago, I felt it was logical that I should be entering menopause. Every woman I knew (that was around my age) was complaining about the mildly uncomfortable to down right severe symptoms they were experiencing. I wondered why I was not experiencing any of these discomforts. I would think to myself, "What is going on anyway? I have never felt better!" About that same time, I had scheduled myself for a routine check-up. Blood and bone density tests were done. When the results came in, the doctor called me. "Well, you're definitely menopausal, Karen. No doubt about it. But it's surprising that you're not experiencing any of the symptoms. Tell me again what you are doing."

I explained that for the past several years I had been consuming a raw plant-based food diet with limited amounts of natural soy products and several ounces of wheat grass per week and had been drinking 3-4 quarts of purified water per day. My physician was very interested and informed me that she had read studies where Asian women who followed traditional eating habits that included substantial amounts of soy experienced little or no menopausal symptoms as well. My results that had come back from the lab had been good enough to warrant exclamation marks next to the results!

The decision to use Hormone Replacement Therapy is one that each woman must make for herself in consultation with a competent health practitioner. I can only tell you that consuming soy products along with consuming mostly raw fruits, vegetables and 3-4 quarts of purified water per day plus eliminating saturated fats, processed foods, sugar, salt, meat and dairy products from my diet appear to have eliminated any suffering I might have incurred from menopausal symptoms.

Health Hint

Coffee and cigarettes deplete naturally occurring estrogen from the body. Do yourself a favor... give them up.

Tofu

My personal preference in soy products is tofu, also known as bean curd. Silken and regular tofu is sometimes labeled as soft, firm or extra firm. Silken tofu is the smoothest in texture. The firmness indicates how much liquid has been extracted from the tofu. I prefer the extra firm form of tofu and have found a wonderful brand that I buy in bulk from my local health food store which can be sliced like cheese. Since I eat no dairy products, this is great to cut in pieces and put on salads. I rarely cook tofu. Since it takes on the flavor of anything it is served with, it deliciously combines with whatever dressing I am using on my salad.

Natural soy products are excellent sources of protein. Protein is necessary for growth and efficient functioning and repair of all tissues and organs. Four ounces of tofu provides the equivalent in protein of two eggs or a medium-sized steak and contains only 120 calories. Combining soy products with non-starchy vegetables or green vegetable salads makes them more readily assimilated by the body. Nuts and seeds are also great sources of protein, but some people find them harder to digest and they are very high in fat.

Most people think they need more protein than they actually do. The truth is that consuming more protein than necessary can actually cause serious problems like overburdening the kidneys. Always be sure to drink plenty of water when eating protein-rich foods.

Other Soy Products

Soy protein as an alternative to meat and dairy products can lower fat intake. Soy products contain an estrogen-like substance. Omega-3 essential fatty acids, calcium, B vitamins and fiber are all found in *whole* soy products. The recommended daily amount is around 25 grams. Soy also has been shown to lower "bad" cholesterol and raise the levels of "good" cholesterol.

There are a number of soy products to choose from. If tofu does not appeal to you, you might try another soy food on the list.

Soymilk
- Soy beverage that can be substituted for milk. Great for those who are Lactose-intolerant.

Soy flour
- This "flour" is a good way to add protein to your baked goods. It can also be used as an egg substitute in baked goods because of its moisture. This can be found in many products. You may already be eating this. Check the labels on foods you have in your cupboard.

Miso
- Fermented soybean paste. This is used in soups and as a seasoning agent.

Tempeh
- Chewy, meat-like substance made from fermented soybeans. It can be used as a meat substitute. It is delicious.

Textured soy protein (TSP)
- Dehydrated soy flour that can be used as a meat substitute or filler in dishes such as meatloaf. Also called Textured Vegetable Protein (TVP).

There are also many soy products that can be used to replace their dairy counterparts such as soy cheese, sour cream, yogurt and ice cream.

Tasty Tofu Tidbits

This is a very delicious way to eat your tofu. I guarantee you will like this one.

- 3 – 4 oz. of extra firm tofu
- Sesame Oil
- Seasoned Rice Vinegar (Lite)
- Toasted Sesame Seeds (optional)

Cut the tofu into bite size cubes and simply drizzle a small amount of the sesame oil and seasoned rice vinegar over the tofu (regular seasoned rice vinegar is high in sodium). Lightly toss the tofu cubes in the oil and vinegar. Sprinkle with toasted sesame seeds.

PART 2

The Mind/Body Connection

CHANGING DIRECTIONS

When I first felt compelled to write this book I wasn't sure where it was coming from. I knew I was constantly being asked questions about how I stayed slim, what I had done to go through menopause without medication, symptoms or discomfort, and how I kept such a consistently high energy level. I knew that I was passionate about telling other women what I had found and how it had changed my life so that they might find the same happiness and peace I had found. I felt that there was no outlet that really addressed these issues like I felt they needed to be addressed. Not from the view of the medical community, but from the perspective of a woman just like each of you. I wanted to supply the information that I could not find years earlier when I was looking for help and present it from the perspective of a loving, caring friend and mentor. I am, as Oprah would put it, "every woman." I represent what every woman can find for herself. This is not a flash in the pan fad. It is not a theory I have come up with. I *know* it works and how it works because I *live* it and successfully maintain the same slim size, an extremely high energy level and have eliminated arthritis, allergies, headaches and other ailments from my life. I have a message that I feel compelled to share. It is a story that doesn't just apply to me. It applies to every woman, no matter what her age. It also dawned on me that it also applies to every man and child. Any person who has a deep desire to change their life and lifestyle for the better can find what I have found. It isn't new and I didn't invent it.

I'm not here to sell you diet products or special formulas. My desire is to contribute to bringing about the peace of mind and elevation of self-esteem that comes naturally with living a food lifestyle that draws our physical, psychological and spiritual aspects together as one harmonious unit. This is something that I was completely unaware of when I started my food lifestyle program. But as I continued to follow my program and make alterations, I experienced more in-depth intuition. I started receiving answers to questions I was seeking in my life that had seemed blocked. I believe that as my body cleared itself of all the toxins and waste, I became more attuned to receiving the answers that were waiting for me.

Fasting has always been universally accepted as a prelude to spiritual connection so it made sense that the more I cleared my body and detoxified it, the more receptive I would be to spiritual connection and awareness. What I was experiencing seemed perfectly natural.

It has been fascinating to observe the new millenium we are moving into. Science and physics are corroborating many of the things that the Bible, other ancient religious teachings and metaphysics have been telling us all along: *we are what we think.* Our thinking overwhelmingly influences our physical, spiritual and psychological reality. It's all interconnected. We may identify food as the problem. We may even find comfort in blaming our parents, our society, our ethnic background or any number of other probable causes for our current state of health. But the bottom line is that we have the choice to change the way we think. That alone will change our lives. Even if you feel, as I did, that you have control over very little of your life, you still have control over the way you eat and the way you think about food. It is symbolic of the way you feel about yourself.

You will find, as I did, that the more you follow this lifestyle food program, the more you will realize that you have control over other things in your life and the more you will want to express that control. I am not talking about control of others. I am talking about feeling that you have the internal power to change not only your external appearance, but that you have the power to change your life. The better care you take of yourself, the better you look and feel. This seems to release a power within you to want to take more calculated risks, to test your potential, to release all that you can be. I will say it again - it is all connected: the physical, psychological and spiritual.

The typical weight-loss diet, as we know it in America, may give us the temporary satisfaction of the loss of a specific amount of pounds, but overwhelming odds are that we will resort to our old ways and the weight will be back. Many times these fad diets may accomplish reducing our bodies to a smaller size dress or pants, but we have depleted our energy and we live in fear that the weight we have shed will return. We are afraid of eating too much and we either deny ourselves or find ourselves bingeing, always afraid that the weight will return and we will be back where we started. Most often, weight is regained and more self-esteem is lost. *Fad dieting is not a solution.*

When we eat what our body naturally desires, we reduce our weight to a level that is perfect and natural for our body and we maintain that weight. Our energy level multiplies. Our physical checkups validate that what we are doing is right. We are able to eat as much as we want without gaining weight. There are no such guarantees with fad diets.

When I first started my food lifestyle change, I gave no thought to the psychological or spiritual ramifications that might take place. That was not my goal. My only goal at that point was to look and feel better and maybe boost my energy level a little. However, after years of this food lifestyle program, I feel that my body has become very cleansed and is quite sensitive and aware of needs that are not *of* the body, but which my body is *a part of.* For example, I now feel a wonderful desire or longing to spend a certain amount of time in solitude, quietly meditating. It may be for only 10-15 minutes in the morning and evening, but my body seems to crave it. I really feel the difference in my body when I don't listen and honor that craving.

THE VALUE OF INNER GUIDANCE

In her article, "The Fat Lady Sings," Natalie Kusz stated, "Food is constantly on any dieter's mind." (*O Magazine*, August 2002) "About that time, it occurred to me that I was succeeding in the world with only part of my brain engaged. While a tenth of it was devoted to school, a tenth devoted to my daughter, and perhaps another tenth to family crises, the other seventy percent was constantly focused on food – the calorie of a grape, the filling bulk of popcorn, the clever use of water as a placebo. I thought to myself, "How much further can I go in the world if I use that seventy percent more wisely?"

Two good indicators of our health are our minds and emotions. It is very important that we realize that the body and the mind work together. When a person is not able to think clearly, is having trouble focusing their attention, experiencing mood swings, lacking energy and enthusiasm and/or feeling depressed, he/she may be feeling the symptoms of a system overloaded with toxins.

In our "just add water and stir" quick-fix society, the promise of instant health, wealth, and success lures us into believing that life altering changes can be accomplished with little or minimal effort and within minimal time constraints. In other words, we think we can get something for nothing. This leads to feelings of ineptness and lowers self-esteem because we fail at these unrealistic expectations every time. We look to the "experts" to tell us what we need to do in every area of our lives. We have been led to believe that we are not intelligent enough to make wise decisions or to take care of ourselves. I am in no way criticizing the medical community. *What I am saying is that we each have an intelligence within ourselves that speaks to us when we listen.* If we are attuned and open, our body gently lets us know exactly what it needs. That is why no one diet is right for everyone. Each individual must determine what is a proper balance for them. The realization of this inner guidance came to me swiftly and harshly through an incident four years ago.

Although my health had been improving miraculously, my right eye had been experiencing some irritation and redness. When it had not dissipated after a period of time, I decided to visit an ophthalmology group. After a few visits, they determined that the eye was "dry" and that I needed punctal plugs inserted in the tear ducts to keep moisture in the eye. It sounded reasonable to me. As I sat in the examining room in preparation for the insertion of the plugs, an incredibly overwhelming urge to leave the office came over me. I am serious when I say that it literally lifted me out of the examination chair. However, my conscious, rational mind logically told me not to be silly. After all, these were experts. What did I know about the treatment of the eye? I had a sick feeling in my stomach, but I forced myself to sit down and wait. The punctul plugs were inserted and almost immediately it was evident that I did not have a dry eye. My eye began to over tear, then overflow in the inner and outer corners of my eye. I was told to go home and that my eye would adjust. Unfortunately it did not.

I subsequently made appointments with one of the top eye surgeons in the country and one of the most prestigious eye clinics in the country. I was told by both that I not only did not have dry eye, but that the fluid integrity was that of a 25-year-old (apparently due to my healthful way of eating). I was also told by both that the standard procedure should have been to observe the eye for several months before taking such a permanent and drastic action. I found that the punctal plugs were made of silicon, therefore, there was no hope of them dissolving. My only options were to live with the condition or have surgery where part of the bone of my nose would be removed and a new tear duct constructed for proper drainage for the eye. I was also informed that this procedure did not work in all cases and that the cost would be around $10,000.

My point here is that your body and subconscious mind speak to you through intuition. You may not always be ready or willing to listen, but their wisdom is always available to guide you to the best choices. I did not listen and I paid a high price. I opted not to have the surgery and, while I am in top health otherwise, I do live with the inconvenience of an over tearing eye, which definitely affects my vision. Had I listened to what my intuition was trying to tell me, had I followed my overwhelming promptings and left the examining room that day, I would not be dealing with this condition today. This experience also made me very aware of the need for at least two opinions (as well as listening to your internal voice) before ever taking any action that could seriously affect your health and life.

It was a high price to pay, but I learned my lesson well. I never, ever make a move in any area of my life without soliciting and listening for that inner guidance. By making this a habit in my life, I have been led to some very wonderful and creative solutions to challenges that have occurred in my life since that time.

GIVE YOURSELF SOME BREATHING SPACE

> *"Breath is the bridge which connects life to consciousness, which unites your body to your thoughts."*
>
> – Thich Nhat Hanh

When speaking of vital nutrients for our body, oxygen is at the top of the list. Oxygen is essential. Our bodies can go without food for weeks. We can even go without water for days. Without oxygen, our life is limited to a few minutes.

It has been said that the average person uses only about one tenth of their total lung capacity. If our body does not get enough oxygen, we feel sluggish and lack energy. If our brain does not get enough oxygen, our thinking does not function properly and we may find ourselves getting irritated easily. All the organs of the body are affected. Lack of oxygen is linked to heart attacks and is considered to be a link to cancer.

The importance of getting enough oxygen cannot be emphasized enough. Especially in the stressful, sedentary world in which we live today where many of us spend the majority of our days confined to cubicles in buildings where the windows are sealed shut.

Deep breathing helps release toxins from our body. It exercises the lungs. It clears the mind. It restores and fills us with calm energy. Deep breathing also has visible, physical benefits such as making the skin glow and smoothing facial lines.

We spend untold hours of our time paying attention to what we eat, but very little thought to seeing that our bodies receive the oxygen it needs to function at its highest level. Since breathing comes naturally, we rarely think about it. Stress and poor posture decrease lung capacity and can make it more difficult to breathe. Breathing into the chest area instead of our abdomen, also known as shallow breathing, limits the amount of oxygen we bring into our body. With shallow breathing, we decrease the circulation of the blood and become tired. When we get caught up in stressful, emotional or rushed activities, we often find ourselves holding our breath. When we do this, we are holding carbon dioxide, a toxin, in our bodies. This toxin then builds up and leads to negative effects on the body. Deep breathing also helps to alleviate feelings of hunger. In many cases this can eliminate self-sabotage for those who are trying to lose weight.

A Simple Breathing Technique:

Tips
- Keep your spine straight.
- Breathe in through the nose, not the mouth. The nose is built to protect the body from unclean substances and extreme cold by "filtering" them out.
- Keep your breathing rhythm consistent.
- Release tension from any muscles by tightening then releasing them.

Technique
- Slowly inhale deeply through your nose for a count of four, taking the breath into the stomach area, not the chest. (Counting while breathing helps take your mind off other things and helps you focus.)
- Hold the breath in the stomach area for a count of four.
- Slowly exhale through your mouth for a count of six until the stomach is completely contracted and the air is completely exhaled.

Do this breathing exercise for about 15 minutes.

The first time you try this exercise you may experience a feeling of light-headedness. Don't be concerned. You are providing your body with extra oxygen that it is not used to receiving. With practice, you will no longer experience this.

Interesting Fact

The animals that live the longest are those who breathe the most slowly.

I do this breathing exercise for 15 minutes each morning. It helps get me focused for the day and provides me with energy. Not the jittery type of energy that one gets from a cup of coffee, but a calm, focused energy. It is a wonderful way to start the day. I also do this exercise for at least 15 minutes before going to bed. Try it. You will be amazed at how quickly you fall off to sleep. No need for sleeping pills!

MENTAL AND SPIRITUAL DETOXIFICATION

> *"A bar of iron costs $5, made into horseshoes its worth is $12, made into needles its worth is $3,500, made into balance springs for watches its worth is $300,000. Your own value is determined also by what you are able to make of yourself."*
> — Author Unknown

It has been reported that the average person thinks approximately 60,000 thoughts per day. When we realize this, it becomes crystal clear that the importance of our mental diet cannot be overstated. Thoughts are continuously running across the horizon of our mind. Take a moment and consciously try to keep thoughts from passing across the panorama of your mind. It is very difficult, if not impossible.

Many people feed their minds a continual diet of toxic thoughts. Toxic thoughts are any thoughts that give power to fear. Fear is the basis of all negative thoughts: anger, insecurity, poverty, hate. When you think that tiny drops of water falling continuously on a solid, impenetrable rock can eventually wear away that rock, it brings into focus how a lifetime of predominantly negative thoughts can destroy and kill even the greatest of talents that dwell within us. Most people lead lives of mental diets filled with the toxic mental foods of "I can't," "I'm not good enough," "I'm not smart enough" or "It won't work." Just for one moment pause and consider what could be accomplished if each of our mental diets consisted of predominantly positive, nurturing thoughts each day. It staggers the imagination. After all, look what miraculous accomplishments we humans are capable of carrying out in this world with predominantly negative attitudes prevailing.

The wonderful news is that just as we can change what we feed our body in order to cleanse it and bring it glowing health, so can we change our mental diet to cleanse our mind and bring us joy, peace and personal success. Our thoughts rule our emotions, our emotions rule our actions and our actions determine the life we live. Therefore, you can see that the thoughts we feed our minds will eventually determine how we live our lives. Just as the foods we eat will eventually determine the health or disease that our body experiences. Look around you. What does your life say about your mental diet?

Let's say you have found that your mental diet could use some improvement, as I found for myself. How do you go about making those changes? This is the question I asked myself long ago. I found that the first step I needed to take was to determine that I *wanted* to change my mental diet and that this was *my* choice, not a choice imposed on me from outside influences. When I stopped pelting myself with *shoulds*, *musts* and *ought tos* and could lovingly say to myself, "The thoughts running through your mind are not bringing you joy, peace or leading you to your best place. Therefore, I am lovingly releasing these toxic thoughts and welcoming only those thoughts that foster strength, love and respect of myself and others," I started to feel my life changing.

This is a process that will not change overnight. After all, this negative thought diet may have been played over and over in your mind for many years. Hypothetically, if some of these negative thoughts began when you were 5-years-old and let's say you are now 45-years-old, it means that you could have played these negative thoughts repeatedly in your mind 21,900,000 times per year for 40 years. In those 40 years you would have run these negative thought recordings over and over approximately 876,000,000 times. Yes, 876 *million* times. Now, do you think that could possibly have an effect on what you believe you can accomplish? You may have established some very habitual ways of thinking. Dialogues may run in your head that you are not even aware of.

Making these changes may appear daunting at first glance. But then, how does that old saying go? "How do you eat an elephant? One bite at a time." (I must make it clear that I have the highest respect for elephants and would never consider eating one!) This is a step-by-step process of change. Just as a computer is programmed, we have programmed our minds to react and respond to certain words, actions and experiences. Now we must re-program our minds.

When we understand the vast power and potential of the mind we are in awe of what is possible. Our conscious mind is our logical, rational mind. Its job is to decipher all input and determine its relationship to our self-preservation. Once our conscious mind makes that determination regarding anything, our subconscious mind accepts this determination as absolute truth. The subconscious accepts anything our conscious mind has accepted as a belief and acts upon that. It does not question the belief but accepts it unconditionally and attempts to fulfill this belief accordingly. This thought is then repeated over and over in our minds. Through the years we program our subconscious to manifest, or create, in our life whatever it is we believe. It doesn't matter if this belief is good or bad, right or wrong, it just works to accomplish the directions that the conscious mind has provided. This is where we experience self-fulfilled prophecies. As Shakespeare so eloquently stated, "A thing is neither good or bad, but thinking makes it so."

When I determined to change my mental diet, I found that spending a certain amount of quiet time alone was a good place to start. This time was spent in just listening to my inner voice and familiarizing myself with my own thoughts. I was not pleased with what I found made up much of my normal, every-day mental diet. So much of it was negative. No wonder I was experiencing so much depression and very little joy. No wonder I felt fatigued and had such low self-esteem. My mind was starving for mental nutrients! I began keeping a journal of my thoughts which helped keep me focused. I would write positive, uplifting thoughts about me, others, my world and the future. I would do this just before retiring at night. I found I was sleeping more peacefully. I would read these thoughts once upon waking. It seemed to jump start my day in a more positive way.

After a short while I felt I needed more. I was feeling more positive. My body was feeling more energetic and was shedding excess pounds. I was consciously working at replacing toxic thoughts with healthy, loving thoughts. It was then that I added a period of meditation to my day.

I never did (and still do not) meditate in the traditional Eastern manner. Although it is a very effective practice, I believe each person must find what is his or her most comfortable way to connect with our inner self and our higher power. There are many books written about meditation and various techniques. If my method does not work for you, look for one that does!

I take 15-30 minutes each morning between 4:30-5:00 a.m. to focus and center my thoughts. It is the most wonderful time of the day. The whole world is quiet and calm. I feel as if I have the world to myself. I also meditate again at the end of the day.

My morning routine:
- Sit with back straight (in bed, in a chair, or on the floor).
- Quietly breathe for several minutes. Inhale through the nose with mouth closed. Hold the breath in the abdomen area — not the chest area — for several seconds. Slowly release the breath through the mouth. Repeat the process for several minutes.
- Tighten and relax the muscles of your body several times to release any tension you are holding in your body. Continue to breathe rhythmically.
- I spend several minutes affirming and mentally visualizing those things I desire in my life with a feeling of joy.
- I give thanks that these or even better things are now appearing or being created for me. I also give thanks for all the good things, people and events that now exist in my life. I individually name many of them.
- I ask what it is I need to know for that day and spend a few minutes just being still and listening for guidance.
- I end by giving thanks for the wonderful, productive day that awaits me.

My evening routine:
- Sit with back straight (in bed, in a chair, or on the floor).
- Quietly breathe and relax the muscles as described in the morning practice.
- I give thanks for the day.
- I ask what I need to learn from my lessons of the day, ask

for guidance and remain quiet for a few minutes.

- I then spend several minutes affirming and mentally visualizing with a feeling of joy those things I desire in my life (just as in the morning practice).
- I give thanks that these things or even better things are now appearing in my life.
- I end by affirming that I will sleep peacefully and that I will be protected and guided by my Higher Intelligence (God or whatever reference you individually make).

I honestly don't know how I got along without these wonderful rituals.

When I started practicing these rituals each day and as my body continued to be cleansed from many years of toxic foods, I was startled as I began to see so many positive, even miraculous, events occur in my life. My depression lifted. I felt very little stress. It was as if they had been lifted off my shoulders. I began feeling that I was always being guided and accompanied by a wonderful, loving friend. My self-esteem began growing and I felt an excitement at the thought of taking on new challenges and risks in my personal and professional life. I began to feel that great possibilities existed all around me. Wonderful coincidences began to happen. Serendipitous events and meetings began to occur.

Our Higher Intelligence has entrusted each of us with the power, potential and life force to determine our own lot in life. When we finally realize this, we feel the responsibility to be an active participant in life rather than settling for sitting back and letting other people or circumstances determine our fate.

I personally began to feel a closeness to God that I had never before experienced. It was not a religious transition, but a gentle awakening of the love and guidance that had been dwelling in me all along. We have been given the great blessing of being able to choose our thoughts *and* beliefs. It cannot be repeated enough that thoughts and beliefs determine emotions, emotions determine actions, and actions determine the life we live.

"According to your faith (belief) be it unto you."
– Matthew 9:29.

By repetition, we can reprogram our negative, toxic thoughts with healthy, empowering thoughts and beliefs. Whenever you find yourself indulging in toxic thoughts, gently acknowledge that you are now releasing these thoughts and replacing them with "nutritious" thoughts. Don't beat yourself up. Accept that it will take some time. I find that I have been practicing this for so long now that when I begin thinking negative thoughts (and it still happens. It is an ongoing process.), it automatically triggers my attention. I then consciously make an empowering statement.

When we speak of affirmations, we are speaking of statements that we make in an assertive, positive way. For example, state "I now desire only those foods that fill me with health and energy," or "I give thanks that I am growing in loving self-confidence each and every day." *Be very careful of the words you use in your everyday life*. Words have great power on the subconscious mind. The subconscious has no sense of humor. It takes everything you say very literally. Emotions also have a large impact on the subconscious, so make sure you state your desires with a feeling of joy, passion and expectation. The subconscious only recognizes *now*, this present moment. It does not function in terms of the past or the future. Therefore, when stating affirmations, don't state things in the future. For example, don't state "My hidden talents *will be* revealed to me and I *will be* guided to my true place in life," but instead state "My hidden talents *are being* revealed to me and I *am now being* guided to my true place in life."

Once your physical body becomes more cleansed internally you will be pleasantly surprised to find that your mind and spirit will follow. You will review your purpose, values, relationships, and all areas of your life. You will become centered in all these areas. Influence from outside sources will have less and less effect on you. You begin to feel very comfortable in your own skin. Many of the toxins that show up as fatigue and depression will begin to leave and you will feel a great lightness and joy. You will appear more attractive to yourself and others. The inner joy radiates to the outer surface. When people start asking you what type of make-up you wear to get that glowing look, you will know for certain that the glow is not a by-product of anything you can apply to your skin. It is a glow that comes from within.

Refuse to accept negative, defeating thoughts. Your subconscious will begin responding in kind, providing you with the kind of life you desire. Your life can be full of interest, joy and accomplishment. Decide what you are going to put your attention on because that is what will grow in your life. *It's your choice.*

Detoxification ACTION STEPS you can take today to cleanse your mind and spirit:
- Listen to motivating audio tapes and CDs.
- Read uplifting material.
- Meditate/Pray.
- Associate with positive, supportive people.
- Keep an open mind to new ideas.
- Spend time in nature gathering the feeling of peace and harmony it provides.
- Treat others well knowing that we are all interconnected.
- Be aware of the words and thoughts you are allowing to enter your subconscious mind.
- Make choices that honor the betterment of yourself and others.
- Express thankfulness today for all the good things in your life.

DETOXIFICATION AND INNER CLEANSING OF THE BODY
Fasting – A Personal Choice
When I used to think of fasting, I visualized chanting monks high on the mountaintops of the Himalayas. That was before I had experienced the power of fasting. Fasting as a form of healing has existed for thousands of years. It has been an accepted procedure used in preparing for spiritual purification by most religions of the world. Even animals are blessed with an inherent knowledge that fasting is the way to heal. When animals become ill, one of the first things they do is cease eating. When this happens, all the energy of the body is free to focus on healing. After all, when the body is digesting food, up to 50% of the body's available energy can be used.

When we fast, we are giving the organs and cells of our bodies a chance to restore and rejuvenate themselves. The process of releasing toxins from our bodies is increased. We often experience an increase in energy, a feeling of rejuvenation, improved sensory perception, weight loss, heightened self-confidence and more mental, emotional and spiritual clarity. Often the flavors of foods are enhanced.

After experiencing periods of fasting over the last several years, I am a firm believer in its benefits. I have taken no medication in the last eight years. I do not even take aspirin. Whenever I find a headache or other bodily disturbance beginning, I try to keep my body in a quiet state, I cut my food consumption drastically and consume large amounts of water (with fresh lemon juice and cayenne) and fresh juices. I have found that within a few hours to a day or so, the symptoms have disappeared. However, I am not a firm believer in strict water fasting or extended fasts. I feel that a day or two of fasting may be beneficial, but that the body needs the ongoing support of nutrients. So, if you are considering beginning a fast, there are a few things you should first consider. The first is the type of fast that is appropriate for you. There are several types of fasts:

Juice Fast	Only fruit or vegetable juices are consumed along with water to supply nutrients that a Water Fast does not.
Mono Fast	Only one type of fruit is consumed for 1 or 2 days.
Modified Fast	Fasting part of the day combined with one light meal.
Water Fast	Only water is consumed. (I do not practice or endorse this type of fast.)

When a person has consumed many toxic and acidic foods over a period of time, there are many toxins that need to be released from the body. A strict fast, such as a water fast, will cause toxins to be released very rapidly. When this happens, the person may experience some rather harsh symptoms such as headaches, fatigue, irritability, dizziness, nausea, restless sleep and bad dreams. You can, however, control the speed with which toxins are released from the body.

The way I fast most often is with the Modified Fast. This is close to my daily routine. I try not to eat anything after about 6:30 pm in the evening. When I rise the next morning, I drink two 16 oz. glasses of room temperature water with the juice of 1/2 to 1 whole fresh lemon squeezed into them. I take 2 tablespoons flax seed oil. I eat nothing except a piece of fruit until noon. This way I am allowing my body a rejuvenation and detoxification period of about 16-18 hours. I wake energetic and this energy carries me through until lunch. I drink another 32 oz. of water 30-60 minutes before lunch.

If this does not appeal to you, try another type of fasting. Choose to take one day every week or two and eat only one type of fruit (Mono Fast). Fruit is very easy to digest. This will give your body a break and will release toxins. You may also choose to take a day or two and consume only fruit and/or vegetable juices (Juice Fast). You may want to dilute the juices with pure water.

Be sure to dry brush while you are fasting to keep the pores of the skin open for the release of toxins. (Dry brushing is discussed later in the chapter) Moderate exercise is important in the release of toxins as well.

As your body becomes cleansed of the accumulated toxins, you will find it easier — and you will actually have the desire — to consume less food. You will love the light, energetic feeling that accompanies the fast. Your thinking will be clearer. Your sense of sight, touch, hearing, smell and taste are enhanced. The natural flavor of foods seems to be more satisfying and you will need little or no salt or flavor enhancers. You begin to enjoy the simple tastes Nature has provided for us. Acid indigestion disappears. I found that I was more aware of my emotions and that I felt more at peace and found a great enjoyment in the mental and spiritual "fasting" of time alone in solitude.

If you choose not to follow any of the fasting suggestions, but simply choose to make changes in your diet, you are still going to make amazing strides in health improvement.

Suggested Fruits (for times of fasting and normal eating):
- Apples
- Bananas
- Cantaloupe (blend this alone, with just a small amount of water)
- Grapes
- Lemon (loosens and releases mucus from the system)
- Mango
- Oranges
- Papaya
- Pears
- Pineapple
- Watermelon

Suggested Vegetables (for times of fasting and normal eating):
- Beets
- Carrots
- Celery
- Cucumber
- Dark Green Leafy Vegetables
- Kale
- Parsley
- Spinach
- Wheat Grass (1 oz. contains the equivalent of 2 lbs fresh vegetables in nutrient value)

WARNING:
Consult your physician before beginning any type of strict water or extended fast.

One of the best things you can do for your body is reduce the amount of calories you are putting into it. We Americans pump far more calories into our body than it needs to run at its most efficient level. Tests done on rodents have shown that when calories were restricted, their life span increased and almost all age-associated physical changes and diseases were slowed down.

Your body is continually in a state of detoxification. In other words, it is continually trying to rid itself of those things that bring ill health. This is especially so during your sleeping hours.

Acid fruits will produce the strongest detoxifying effect. Starting your day with a glass of warm water with fresh-squeezed lemon will help intensify the detoxifying process of the liver and has mild laxative properties.

Fiber & Colon Cleansing

While people are becoming increasingly aware of the importance of consuming nutritious foods, few realize that the inability to eliminate wastes from our bodies results in toxic, rotting matter in the colon, which is the large intestines. This is the last portion of your body's food processing chain.

The "Big 3" in this area, *water, fiber and moderate exercise*, all play a vital role in proper elimination of waste from our bodies.

Dr. Bernard Jensen, D.C., Ph.D., Nutritionist, uses a great analogy: "Imagine what would be the result of a pump failure in a city's sewer system. What would happen if the pipes got all plugged up with some unmovable material so that the system failed to move waste? It wouldn't take very long before a crises developed and a huge sanitation problem would threaten health and society."

It has been reported that a person consuming the typical American diet can hold up to eight meals of undigested food in their system, while a person on a high fiber diet will hold only about three meals. Meats, fats and sugar in the diet slow the time from the ingestion of food to its elimination from the body in the form of a bowel movement. The fact is, it can take from two days to nearly one week for this type of diet to complete its process of elimination from the body! In fact, waste matter can sit in your colon for weeks and even months, poisoning your entire system. Compare this to one day in cultures where high fiber diets are consumed.

When this decomposing matter sits in the body for two days to a week, opportunities for exposure to carcinogenic substances and harmful bacteria is greatly multiplied and blocks the intestine from absorbing the necessary nutrients. In the September 1982 issue of *Lancet*, it was reported that rates of death from cancer and all other causes were approximately three times higher for men in the lowest category of dietary fiber intake than for those in the highest category.

If you are drinking eight 8 oz. glasses of water per day, consuming plenty of fiber rich foods and getting moderate exercise, but still find that you are experiencing constipation or other disorders of the bowel, this may be a sign of some other disorder in your body. If this happens, you should contact your physician.

There are some individuals who have a low tolerance to fiber. This may result in gas, bloating and pain. The average person, however, should respond very efficiently to added fiber.

Adequate dietary fiber and plenty of water is absolutely necessary if we are to maintain health at an optimal level. A daily fiber intake of 30-50 grams per day is recommended. Dietary fiber can be divided into two basic types: soluble and insoluble. The soluble type dissolves in water, the insoluble type does not. Both provide bulk in the large intestine and encourage regular elimination from the bowels.

Water Soluble Fiber	Insoluble Fiber
Oat Bran	Wheat Bran
Fruits High in Pectin (apple, peach, currant, plum)	Whole Grain Products (Oatmeal, Brown Rice, etc.)
Psyllium Husk (a natural water soluble fiber)	Fruits with Edible Seed
Legumes	Vegetables

At this point, it appears that soluble fiber has added benefits to the body as opposed to the insoluble type. One major benefit is the apparent ability to help lower blood cholesterol levels. (A word of warning: if you are taking any drug to control your cholesterol level, consult your physician before attempting to alter your dosage or discontinue its use). An additional benefit is the stimulation of the secretion of pancreatic enzymes.

A Word About Colon Irrigation

Along with the consumption of a high fiber diet, many people now choose to self-treat themselves with colon irrigations or to have professional colonics. Colonics remove wastes from the entire large intestine. There appear to be no harmful side effects to this process. However, these treatments can stir up dormant toxins in the mucous layers of the colon. A small amount of these toxins may be re-absorbed by the system. If this happens, you may experience some temporary symptoms such as nausea, headaches or a dizzy feeling. This typically means that there is more cleansing necessary.

Enemas are different from colonics because they only flush out the bottom portion of the colon removing the new waste that is present. Use warm spring water or water that has had the chlorine filtered out. You may add strong boiled coffee which stimulates the peristaltic contractions, contains acids that help remove mucous, cleanse the colon wall and helps to reduce the bile level in the liver. If you are sensitive to caffeine, you may want to use lemon juice instead. Again, you may choose just to use plain, warm spring water.

Let's Address the Laxative Issue

The use of laxatives to cleanse the colon is not recommended. These can actually irritate the colon. Continued use of laxatives wears out the bowel muscle and may cause it to fail to function in its normal and proper manner. Some laxatives contain harsh substances that may be absorbed into your system.

Remember the 3 important Do's regarding Colon Cleansing:
1. Eat High Fiber Foods
2. Drink eight 8 oz. glasses of water each day
3. Get moderate exercise (walking, etc.)

High Fiber Foods
Fresh Fruits
Fresh Vegetables
Legumes

Dry Brush Body Detox

This tradition is said to go back hundreds, maybe even thousands, of years and is attributed to the Scandinavian countries.

The skin is the body's largest organ. Toxins must be allowed to exit the body through the skin pores or the other detoxification organs will be overburdened. In order for these toxins to be released through the skin, the pores must remain unclogged. By gently brushing the skin we slough off the old dead cells. As an added benefit circulation is increased. Dry brushing also helps reduce those unsightly fatty pockets (cellulite) that gather under the skin.

You will want to purchase a natural bristle brush. These can be picked up at any health food, bath, or drug store. Use a dry brush on dry skin. Start at the toes and fingers and always use gentle brushing strokes in the direction of the heart. The delicate skin of the face and neck should be avoided when brushing. It is very important that you brush in the underarm and the inner thigh areas to get the circulation flowing around the lymph nodes. These lymph nodes assist the body in filtering and eliminating potentially harmful or toxic substances from the body. They have no circulation system of their own, unlike the blood system which has the heart as its pump.

I always do this just before showering. It feels wonderful and gets those toxins moving out of your system.

STRESS AND DIET

Do you feel strung out and anxious before you even get to work or start your day? Most people don't realize the connection between stress and the food they put into their bodies. There are foods that can increase your anxiety level and others that can soothe jangled nerves.

If you are serious about lowering your stress level, incorporate a diet that is low in refined sugar, fats, starches and protein. Forget the morning biscuits, cake and cookies and white, doughy bread toast. Instead go for raw vegetables, fresh or dried fruits, unsalted nuts or sprouted grain breads. Purified water and natural fruit juices aid calming of nerves.

There are a couple of substances that need to be discussed

specifically. These substances can actually trigger stress reactions because of the effects they have on our body's nervous system.

Caffeine can increase our heart rate and blood pressure and make the nervous system very reactive. Anxiety and depression can be triggered by habitual consumption of coffee, cola or tea. (These drinks can also cause loss of important body fluids since they are diuretics). The negative effect of caffeine provokes insulin release and may, in fact, enhance the storage of what is eaten as fat.

Sugar is another culprit to be especially aware of. There are numerous studies that show the decreases in the immune system functions following sugar consumption. The average American consumes approximately 150 pounds of sugar each year.

Moderate exercise and sufficient rest also have a positive effect on stress reduction.

GOOD HEALTH IS A LAUGHING MATTER

"Humor is mankind's greatest blessing."
– Mark Twain

It is now generally accepted that the mind, body and spirit are connected. How we think has a great effect on how we feel. When we are happy and feel joyous we release healthy chemicals in our bodies. When we are unhappy, we actually suppress our immune system.

Norman Cousins wrote a book concerning the medicinal benefits of laughter. He found great relief from the pain of cancer through his self-prescribed laughter medicine. How many times do you laugh in a day? Various studies report that children laugh on the average anywhere from 100 – 400 times each day. An adult, on the other hand, is reported to laugh an average of a meager 5 – 20 times a day. Regardless of which study is the most accurate, the overwhelming finding is that there is a huge discrepancy between the number of times children laugh per day versus adults. Many adults have forgotten to look for the humorous, playful or amusing events in life.

Children always view the world with a sense of wonder.

Every raindrop is amazing. They are never in such a hurry that they can't take time out to experience the world around them. However, we learn early in our culture that success in life and our image is no laughing matter. We learn that to be taken seriously, we must display seriousness, even sternness. It is undeniable that a certain amount of seriousness is appropriate in our lives. However, we have lost sight of the fact that laughter is healthy. It is a great stress reliever. Instead of holding those worries inside like a pressure cooker, how much better it is when we are able to diffuse them through the use of appropriate humor. Instead of filling our bodies full of processed and lifeless "comfort" foods in an attempt to alleviate our stress or worries, how much better to be able to release comforting, healing endorphins throughout our systems through laughter.

A sense of humor makes a very important contribution to a healthy body. Laughing boosts the immune system. It enhances the release of endorphins. Toxins are released from our systems. Our cardiopulmonary functions are enhanced.

As you start this new way of life, it is very important that you are able to laugh at yourself. When you can do that, you are actually treating yourself in a kinder, gentler manner. You don't expect the impossible of yourself. Whenever you start something new, there is a certain period of learning and familiarizing you must go through. There will be times that you will slide back a little. It's ok. I still do too on occasion. This is a continual learning process. Evaluate what caused you to slide backwards. Record it in your journal as a learning tool. Realize that your self-knowledge is growing. Then move on.

After having practiced this program of eating for many years, I can say without hesitation that a light, joyous feeling is a natural by-product of this way of life. It is my opinion that it is a result of having a clean system free of toxins. The body is free to provide you with boundless energy instead of being immersed in a continual battle against toxic wastes in your system which constantly threaten your health.

Remember, as in all things, how you respond to the events around you is your choice.

Choose to:
- Look for something humorous in today's occurrences.
- Seek out people who are able to laugh.
- Laugh at least 10 times today and then increase that to 11 times tomorrow.
- Observe children. Recapture that wonder.
- Start watching more funny movies.
- Read more cartoons.
- Laugh at yourself!

The following poem was provided in the 8/19/02 issue of *Healthwell* and was attributed to James Greenblatt, MD, of Newton, Massachusetts. I loved it and thought you would too:

10 Warning Signs of Good Health
1. Persistent sense of humor
2. Chronic positive expectations; tendency to frame events in a constructive light
3. Episodic outbreaks of joyful, happy experiences
4. Sense of spiritual involvement
5. Tendency to adapt well to changing conditions
6. Rapid response to and recovery from stress and repeated challenges
7. Increased appetite for physical activity
8. Tendency to identify and communicate feelings
9. Repeated episodes of gratitude and generosity
10. Continuing presence of support network

Remember: laughing 100 times is equal to 10 minutes on the rowing machine or 15 minutes on the exercise bike!

BECOMING CONNECTED

For years I just started and stopped diet and lifestyle programs without a plan or any focus. I always just hoped things would work. In retrospect, I can see that this method of approach is about as effective as attempting to build my dream home with only a pile of lumber and a can of nails.

In the past we women traditionally have lived so much of our lives trying to support others, that many of us have never taken the time to know and understand our own mind/body/ spirit connection. We have had no idea what we want out of life, what our talents are or what our purpose is. Many of us have devoted our lives to seeing that our husbands and children are supported and encouraged in pursuing their dreams. This is a wonderful and worthwhile goal, but many women have followed this to the exclusion of their own dreams and fulfillment. It is my belief that in many instances food is used to fill the hollow spaces of those unfulfilled dreams.

After I had become separated in my marriage and was attempting to build a life on my own, it suddenly became very clear that I had nurtured all those around me but I had not nurtured myself. I had no idea what I wanted to do with my life or what my purpose might be. I was blindly applying for any job that had an opening, not looking for something that would fit my unique needs and talents. I was lost. But then a small incident occurred that had a huge impact on my way of thinking. One evening, during a lull in the conversation, an acquaintance posed a few questions to me. The questions were neither difficult nor too personal. They were questions as simple as, "What are your three favorite books?" "What are your three favorite foods?" You get my drift. I sat there at a loss for words. I, literally, could not name three things in any of the categories that my acquaintance had asked about.

Over the years I had lost touch with myself. I could not answer the most basic questions about who I was. This shook me to my foundation. After all, if I didn't know the answer to simple questions about who I was, then how could I possibly know what I wanted out of life or what my purpose was? It shook me so much that I went home that very night and sat up for hours asking myself every question I could think of and trying to give three answers to each question.

Since that revealing night, I have made it a practice to continually notice and be aware of what delights my senses, mind and spirit. I believe they are Divine clues to our work and purpose here. It has been and continues to be a very rewarding journey. I continue to learn more about myself each day. An added benefit is that I have become reacquainted with myself. I began remembering those things that gave me delight as a child. These, I believe, are clues as well. I began appreciating myself more and finding myself being more creative in my life. I have also made it a point to ask other women questions similar to those I was asked. So very often I find that when I present a woman with these questions, she is stunned at how little she knows about herself.

Whether or not you are able to name your three favorite foods is not important. But by starting with simple questions like these, you begin stimulating your mind. You begin to discover what makes you sing and what brings out your passion.

YOUR JOURNALS – DON'T LEAVE HOME WITHOUT THEM

Keeping a journal is invaluable. Layer by layer, it will truly reveal the "essence of you." It can reveal blocks and habitual patterns that may be holding you back. It can reveal your true values. It can alert you to areas of your life that need to be reexamined. It can reveal hidden talents, strengths, potential and purpose. A journal is a wonderful, silent friend who you can share your most personal thoughts with and never have to be concerned about reactions of any kind.

I suggest that you keep two journals: a food journal and a personal journal.

Food Journal

This is a record of all the foods you consume, the hours of the day you are consuming them and how you feel 15-30 minutes after eating them. It's purpose is to learn about food combining, maintaining a stable blood sugar level, what foods give you energy, deplete energy, make you fatigued or are mood altering. Include in your journal any feelings you have related to eating. For example, if you are feeling a binge coming on, sit down and write what you are feeling and try to determine where it is coming from. What is happening in your life right now? Can you deal with it in a more effective manner than binge eating? Believe me, this journal is well worth the investment of your time. You will become more attuned to hearing what your body is trying to communicate to you.

Example of a Food Journal Page:

Week: _____ – What I Found Out About Me

What Worked	What Didn't Work
1. I felt light and energetic after eating these foods: Time of Day:	1. I experienced a feeling of gas, indigestion or bloating after eating these foods: Time of Day:
2. I felt the most centered and calm after eating these foods: Time of Day:	2. I experienced feelings of anxiety, headaches or irritability after eating these foods: Time of Day:
3. My energy level seemed to be evenly sustained the longest after eating these foods: Time of Day:	3. My energy level seemed to be low or erratic after eating these foods: Time of Day:
4. I noticed relief from (any previous symptom) after eating these foods:	4. I experienced constipation after eating these foods:
The foods I am finding make me feel the best are:	**The foods that I am discovering don't work well with my body are:**
Notes:	**Notes:**

Personal Journal

We have discussed the importance of a food journal previously. You should also begin a personal journal. I carry a small 3x5 journal with me. Begin writing any and all things that move you, interest you or even disturb you. It's all part of the process of becoming whole. Keep in mind that many of the ways we eat, act or believe are a result of habit, tradition, cultural background, social pressure or mass media programming. Reexamine your entries. Determine if they are really nurturing you in mind/body/spirit, or do you just perform them according to rote. A few months later when you go back over the information, you will be astounded to see how you have progressed and what you have discovered about yourself. It is the best gift anyone could give you. And you can give it to yourself.

I began keeping a journal years ago when was I going through some very painful experiences. As I look back over the journals from this time period, I am amazed at what I learn about myself, my values, and how I have grown. Journals are wonderful tools for growth measurement.

Your personal journal is a record of your personal feelings about *everything*. You will reveal and uncover the real essence of you. When you sit down, don't worry about what you will write, just start writing. Write whatever comes into your head. No one is going to read this but you. This is your personal, private world. Put down your feelings. Ask yourself probing questions about your values. What are you willing to accept in your life? What will you no longer accept? What kind of relationships do you want in your life? What talents have you neglected? I find that writing very early in the morning is the best time for me. For whatever reason, once I start writing, the words just seem to pour out. I can promise you that after a few months time, you will be able to go back over your entries and you will be amazed at how your life has changed or how you have changed and your life has altered as a natural result of your changes. You may clearly see behavioral patterns that you did not even know existed previously. I began to see how I had made some of the same bad choices over and over again in my life, but just kept expecting my life to improve. My personal journal allowed me to see the consequences of my past choices and aided me in laying a firm foundation for my new, productive life.

Sometimes we become aware not only of ineffective behaviors, but also of negative thinking patterns that have kept us stuck. The journal can help us get out of our own way so that we can accomplish the goals we desire. Is your journal filled with words such as *should, ought to, have to, never, always* and so on? You may be blocking your own progress. Start replacing some of the negatives with positive affirmations about your progress such as "With each new day I am taking better and better care of myself. I desire only those foods that bring me health and energy." Or "I continually attract positive supportive people into my experience." It can be anything that is life affirming and uplifting. Just be sure to make the statement in the present tense and state it positively.

Your subconscious is highly suggestive when you are in a very relaxed or sleepy state. If you are trying to resolve an issue, just before going to sleep write the question down and give clear instructions to your subconscious to answer it. You may be very surprised to receive the answer to your question within the next few days and in ways you had not expected.

When we begin to release toxins and are cleansed physically, mentally and spiritually, we begin to realize how very powerful our mind is and what a powerful tool our journal can be in the reshaping of our lives and accomplishing of our goals.

The following questions will help you to get started. I will not include favorite food questions and the like. You can handle that yourself. The following questions are to start you looking at your responses to life and help you determine where you want to make changes:

1. What is your definition of commitment?
2. What would your life be like right now if you were living the life you dream of for yourself? What are you willing to commit to in order to reach that goal?
3. What benefits are you looking for as you enter this lifestyle change?
   Examples:
   • Reach ideal weight

- Be free from pain
- Have more energy
- Effectively control stress
- Live longer
- Feel more in control of the areas of your life
- Higher self-esteem
- Live medication free
- Find purpose and meaning
- (Add your own desired benefit)

4. What and who in your life is toxic/healthy? How are they affecting your life?
5. What are the five most important values in life to you?
6. What is your definition of success?
7. What negative influences are keeping you blocked? Are you willing to change them?
8. What do you see as the payoff for making a change in your lifestyle now?
9. Do you feel that you are not only worthy of giving, but also of receiving?
10. Do you focus on your strengths or your weaknesses?
11. How would you define yourself? Your body?
12. Do you feel you have a valuable purpose to play in society?
13. What negative behaviors are you willing to release?
14. What new life-affirming behaviors are you willing to embrace?
15. When you look in the mirror, do you see your best friend or your worst enemy?

Personal Commitment Statement

After considering the above questions, find a quiet place and write a *Commitment Statement* for yourself. It doesn't have to be lengthy. Just write a couple of clear, concise paragraphs. It is important to put your intentions in writing, then sign and date it. This indicates to your subconscious that you mean business. Re-read this statement each day so the subconscious absorbs the belief and reality of your commitment.

My Personal Commitment Statement

_____

_____

_____

_____

_____

_____

_____

_____

_____

_____

Signature: _____ Date: _____

Just a Thought

5 lbs. does not seem like much, does it? Do this the next time you are at the supermarket: walk back to the meat counter and look at a 5 lb. roast. Lift it up and carry it around for a couple of minutes. Now consider the stress you are putting on your body by carrying those extra 5 lb. (or however many lbs.) around everywhere you go, 24 hours a day. You can choose to change your life today.

MAKING A START

"As a being of power, intelligence, and love, and the lord of your own thoughts, you contain within yourself that transforming and regenerative agency by which you may make yourself what you will."
– James Allen

One of the first things people say to me when discussing making a change in their life and their eating style is "I don't even know where to start." So... can we talk?

The first and most basic place to start is with **choice**. You must make the conscious choice that you want, and I mean *really* want, a better life. Are you willing to not merely talk the talk, but actually walk the walk? When you finally come to the realization that you are continuously choosing, you realize that even not making a choice is actually making a choice. It is a choice to do nothing or continue doing those things that have not worked in the past. So why not make a choice this very minute to start taking care of and treating yourself with the respect you deserve?

The second concept to consider is **responsibility**. Yes, that's right. *You* are responsible for your own health and happiness. This means there will be no blaming others, your past conditioning or anything else for your situation. In no way do I mean you should dismiss any circumstances which may have occurred in your past. But to get you to a new place of health, happiness and success, you must move past these circumstances and create a "wellness way of living." Only you can do this. *You* are responsible.

The third concept to consider in starting this wellness way of life is realizing that **nature governs itself by laws**. These laws are eternal and never changing. They pertain to everyone. There are no exceptions. There is no favoritism or partiality shown. Nature's byword is *balance* and it is to that end that we strive. When we ignore Nature's laws, we pay the price. Plain and simple.

The fourth concept to consider is that **the mind, body and** *spirit all work together.* When you affect a change in the body, you also affect the mind and vise versa. They are interconnected. When we are serious about changing our lives, it is necessary that we consider that each of these areas will be affected and will call for nourishment.

It is a good idea to take a few minutes to get clear in your mind where you are mentally. By asking yourself a few questions, you may find that you actually have a better idea of where to start than you thought you had. Give yourself the gift of taking a few moments now to answer the following questions:

1. Do I feel I have the power to make choices in my life? In my attitudes?
2. Am I willing to be open to taking risks to move into a new, more fulfilling and rewarding lifestyle?
3. Am I giving my valuable energy to people and situations from the past?
4. Am I willing to be flexible along the way?
5. Do I believe deep down that I am worthy of reaching my goals?
6. Do I believe I deserve to be healthy and full of joy?
7. Am I giving myself big enough goals?
8. Am I willing to let go of negative thoughts that have blocked my success in the past?
9. Do I truly want to succeed?

Remember: we all have to start from where we are.

THE PLANT-BASED FOOD LIFESTYLE

While the basics of this lifestyle are the same for all: man, woman or child. We must remember that each of us is coming from a different place mentally, spiritually, and physically. That is why fad diets are just that… fads. They don't last because they don't address the needs of the individual. These diet programs herd everyone into a mass group and provide them with a "one size fits all" plan. We've all had the experience of trying on the "one size fits all" clothing. Maybe the clothing actually fits one in one hundred persons well. It's the same for fad diet programs.

In this book I will lay out the fundamentals of Nature's laws on weight loss and stabilization, regaining and retaining health, developing clarity of mind, and opening oneself to the innate guidance that is in each one of us. However, from these basic guidelines we must observe and discover what works best for us. One person may feel better consuming more fruit. Another person may feel better consuming more vegetables than fruit. Although nuts are good for us, one person may find them harder to digest than another. So you see what I mean. Based around the fundamentals, we will each develop a plan that works for us. The beauty of this plan is that after you have been following it for a while, you will discover that you are beginning to know yourself in a way you have never known before. You will discover that this way of eating is *meant* to last a lifetime. You will find out what gives you energy and what depletes your energy. You will find out when you are most productive and when you are not. You will find what affects your moods and your sleeping patterns. You will find which foods work together in your body and which don't. You will not need any outside "experts" telling you what you should and shouldn't do. The only expert you need to rely on is your body. Believe me, it will let you know what is working and what is not. When you treat your body well, it will love and repay you in the most wonderful and rewarding ways.

Some of you will be prepared to go headfirst into this program. You are ready to apply all the fundamentals and move ahead as rapidly as possible. Others will choose to enter more slowly, examining each principle for its truth. Whichever way you choose to enter this new lifestyle is not important. That you actually make the conscious decision to change your life for the better and enter this way of living is where the true importance lies.

It is my great hope that you choose to apply all the principles and information provided in this book starting today. I know them to be true. Following this food program for the last eight years has changed everything in my life: mentally, physically and spiritually. The changes are powerful, positive and enduring. But if all you decide to do right now is to eliminate white, refined sugar and flour products from you diet or to drink one quart of water a day or to eat one meal per day of raw fruits or vegetables, you are making a positive step toward wellness. I believe that the more you do, the more you will want to do.

This book will provide you with informational tables, lists of recommended foods (and foods that are not recommended) and information on combining different types of foods. I have provided only a few recipes because I only rely on a few. I keep my meals very simple to allow my body the most ease in the digestion process. There are many good books on vegetarian and raw food recipes available in health food and book stores, libraries, and on the Internet.

PART 3

The Living Food Lifestyle Basics

WHY RAW FOODS?

One of the greatest benefits of consuming raw foods is the cleansing of toxins and wastes from the body. Fruits are natural cleansers. Vegetables are natural restorers and builders. Raw food has a rejuvenating effect on the entire body. All functions of the organ systems, including the skin, improve noticeably. Studies conducted on consumption of raw foods have reported extremely positive results regarding rejuvenation and even reversal of the aging processes. The skin takes on a youthful glow and feel.

Healthy Hint

Digestion uses about 50% of your vital energy to break down the food you eat. The remaining energy is available for every other life operating process. Therefore the lighter you eat, the more vital energy is available to work on other processes such as healing.

Before discussing the benefits of following a living or raw plant-based food lifestyle, we should define what living foods are. Living foods contain enzymes. Enzymes not only digest food, but also regulate almost every function that goes on in your body. Nature has planned well for our bodies. Every plant-based raw food contains all the enzymes needed to digest that particular food. These enzymes are activated by your saliva and the moisture and heat which is produced during chewing.

Research has shown that all enzymes are virtually destroyed when food is cooked at approximately 118°F. This renders the food lifeless. So what happens then? Because that food has no enzymes of its own to digest it, the body must borrow enzymes from other parts of the body to digest this lifeless food. The more the body's enzymes must be used for digestion, the less there are for running the body and performing its necessary functions. As we age, the number of enzymes in our body naturally decreases. Antioxidants have a tougher time doing their job if there are not sufficient enzymes.

Canned and processed foods have the same effect on the body. The body is forced to provide enzymes from other vital functions to digest this dead food. Food additives can also destroy enzymes. Take a moment to look at your average daily consumption of food. What do you eat for breakfast, lunch, dinner and snacks? How much of it is empty of enzymes? It may astound you. Look at the number of wrappers in your garbage. It has been said that we can tell how destructive our diet is by the amount of food packaging and wrappers we discard. Most of these packaged items are pumped full of additives, preservatives, chemicals and dyes. When you discard a processed food, you add to the "waste heap". They just sit there and pile up because they are usually non-biodegradable. When you discard the remains of a raw plant-based food, you feed the ongoing process of life. The remains are biodegradable and decompose. They return to the earth in order to provide nutrients to another plant.

Most people today assume that cooked food is just the natural way of eating. However, the book *Over Fifty, Looking Thirty* by Nina Anderson and Howard Peiper, goes into an explanation that humans are the only species that cook their food. Humans are also the only species that suffer from widespread diseases and sicknesses. The authors go on to state that research has shown white blood cells double or triple after eating a cooked meal. This is because the immune system interprets this dead food that is being ingested as an enemy and it sends troops (white blood cells) to fight it. Enzymes are then released from these cells to digest this food. This is not the job of the immune system. If this situation is ongoing, the body may create physical reactions which we know as food allergies. When a diet is continually deficient in enzymes, the immune system is weakened because the infection fighting enzymes are now having to digest this food.

T. Colin Campbell, Ph.D. of Cornell University states that "the evidence includes the recommendations that heating of many kinds of foods is known to produce certain chemicals that have long been known to be carcinogenic under certain conditions. These chemicals include the heterocyclic amines and polyaromatic hydrocarbons."

If we are to enjoy optimal health and energy we need to be consuming approximately 75% raw plant-based food in our diets. In the book *Raw Energy*, authors Leslie and Susannah Kenton state that a "vast quantity of evidence exists showing that the high raw diet — a way of eating in which 75% of your foods are taken raw — cannot only reverse the bodily degeneration which accompanies long-term illness, but retard the rate at which you age, bringing you seemingly boundless energy and even make you feel better emotionally." I have found over the years that the more raw fruits and vegetables you eat, the more your appetite for them increases.

ENZYMES

Let me introduce you to some of your best friends. They work tirelessly to help provide you with optimum health. They are on the job night and day. Without their continual efforts we would not be alive. However, few people are even aware of their existence. These friends are called enzymes.

Our bodies have many, many types of enzymes. Enzymes are protein molecules and are absolutely necessary to every chemical function in our bodies such as digestion, healing, and so on. They are found in the pancreas, liver, salivary glands, intestines and stomach. They are also found in raw plant-based foods.

To explain how enzymes work, let's take a look at a piece of fruit. The ripening process is actually caused by enzymes at work. As the fruit ripens, you are observing the enzymes going through their process of breaking down the fruit and digesting it. This process makes it very easy for this fruit to be digested and pass through our bodies.

Enzymes can only be found in living foods. Let's say you have decided to consume your fruit by drinking juice. Be sure the juice is fresh and unpasteurized. Pasteurized juice has a longer shelf life, but the heating process of pasteurization has destroyed the enzymes. Pasteurization robs your body of the chance to use the enzymes that nature had lovingly put in that fruit to aid your body in the digestion process.

Your body will do its best for you, but if you are eating improperly, it must now work harder, often causing a hardship on the liver and pancreas. Worker enzymes must be called from other crucial functions to perform this work. So many times we curse our bodies for not performing in the manner we expect when in actuality we have been responsible for putting our bodies through so much abuse while they tirelessly continue to try to function, heal and adapt.

Our bodies have three primary types of digestive enzymes. Each one has a special function:

ENZYME	FUNCTION
Protease	To break down proteins
Amylase	To break down carbohydrates and starch
Lipase	To break down fats

As touched upon earlier, when we cook foods at temperatures of approximately 118°F and above, we destroy the enzymes that are found in live, fresh foods. The life or energy giving force is gone. These enzymes were built into raw plant-based foods by Nature as a means of providing proper and complete digestion in our bodies. They even contain the fiber to carry the wastes out of our systems. When these enzymes are no longer available due to the cooking process, enzymes have to be borrowed from other activities going on in the body in order to digest these foods. Our body only produces a limited number of its own enzymes during a lifetime. Without enzymes, these minerals, vitamins and hormones cannot do their work. As these metabolic enzymes become depleted, we set in motion the aging process and the body begins to deteriorate.

In the February 2001 issue of *Living and Raw Foods* it is reported that "A youth of 18 may produce amylase levels 30 times greater than those of an 85 year old person." As we get older it is vitally important to our continued good health — not to mention looks — that we provide our bodies fresh, energy giving foods packed with life force: enzymes.

When enzymes must work on processed or cooked foods it takes longer to pass through the body. This causes fermentation and the creation of toxins. Many people just don't know or connect the fact that the toxins lurking and lounging in their systems for extended periods of time are contributing significantly to:

- arthritis
- allergies

- irritability
- headaches
- irregularity
- nervousness
- skin problems
- feelings of fatigue
- recurring infections
- intestinal discomfort

In their book *Over 50 Looking 30!* Nina Anderson and Howard Peiper state: "When the white blood cells are continually elevated due to a diet in enzyme deficient foods, the immune system is weakened because the infection fighting enzymes are now trying to digest food!" They continue "Every raw food contains exactly the right amount and types of enzymes to digest that particular food." This is a strong clue that we are meant to consume our foods in a live, raw state.

Some of the richest sources of enzymes are listed below. Try to include them in your diet. Enzymes are available in tablet form and may be purchased at any reputable health food store. I do not personally take enzyme supplements because raw food makes up the majority of my diet. However, for those who still consume many cooked foods, these foods and/or supplements might be something you want to add to your diet to aid in the digestion process.

- Papaya
- Pineapple
- Sprouts
- Chlorophyll (plentiful in sprouts and greens)

THE ACID/ALKALINE CONNECTION

A very important part of this program is understanding the body's acid/alkaline connection.

According to *The BiologyReport,* University of Arizona, January 19, 1999, "The normal range for blood pH is 7.35-7.45." That is a slightly alkaline range. Anything above 7.0 is alkaline and anything below 7.0 is acidic. When we eat foods, the residue left from the metabolism of the foods is like ash. It can be alkaline or acidic. Most of the foods consumed by the American public, such as meat, dairy and grain products, are highly acidic. When this acid residue is left in the system the body will try to compensate by pulling alkaline substances out of the cells to neutralize the acids. This leaves the cells in an acid state known as *acidosis*. When this happens, the body's abilities to absorb minerals and other nutrients, repair damaged cells, and detoxify heavy metals is decreased. The body becomes more susceptible to fatigue, illness and disease. Research is finding that there is clearly a connection between the pH level of the blood and the level of disease in the body. Chronic inflammation, congestion, allergies, fatigue, recurrent infections, cancer, cardiovascular disease, diabetes and other disease states appear in people whose bodies are in an acidic state.

White flour and sugar products, soft drinks, coffee, artificial sweeteners and many medications are also extremely acid forming and add to this toxic state in our body.

To function at its optimum level, our body should be slightly alkaline. Alkaline forming foods include fruits, leafy greens, vegetables, lentils, nuts and seeds. (Note: nuts and seeds can be somewhat acidic as well and should be eaten in moderation.)

Acid forming foods include meat, poultry, eggs, grains, legumes and fish. Some of the highest acid residue producing foods are also very mucus producing. Thick mucus is the body's way of trying to protect itself from the toxins that acid producing foods generate.

I try to eat as many alkaline forming foods as possible and limit consumption of acid forming foods. Aim for a 60% alkaline/40% acid ratio to start with and make your goal 80% alkaline/20% acid or higher. This may take some adjustment on your part, but you will find the rewards well worth it. You will see improvements in your health that you did not even anticipate. As I had stated earlier, since implementing this program in my life, the arthritis, allergies, ulcers and cold in my hands and feet have disappeared and have never returned. See Appendix for a list of both alkaline and acid forming foods. Use these lists to help you make your selection when planning your meals.

A diet of 70-80% alkaline and 20-30% acid will keep our body in good health. According to Health Freedom Resources of Clearwater, Florida, the average American diet consists of 20-30% alkaline foods while the optimal diet should consist of at least 70-80% alkaline foods. They go on to state that it is not unusual for the average American to go 7-14 days without eating ANY alkaline foods.

Three Culprits in the Acid/Alkaline Story

Meat. Let's face it — flesh begins to decompose the moment an animal dies. Bacteria, uric acid and even parasites are frequently present. *Fact.* Humans have the tooth formation for leaf crushing, not flesh tearing. *Fact.* Even the leanest of meats is relatively high in fat. *Fact.* Research has linked cancer to animal foods.

America's obsessive, misinformed idea that you can only get protein from meat is just that — *misinformation.* Traditional sources of protein such as fatty beef and other red meats are loaded with saturated fats and cholesterol, which contribute to heart disease. In fact, in an article on soy products that appeared in the *American Journal of Clinical Nutrition* stated: "It can be concluded that, except for premature infants, soy protein can serve as a sole protein source in the human body."

Dairy Products. We are still being told that milk is good for us. Fortunately, many people are moving away from this idea. In the December 16, 2002 issue of *AD Health Articles*, Dr. Michael Klaper, M.D. is quoted as saying, "It's not natural for humans to drink cow's milk. Human milk is for humans. Cow's milk is for calves… Cow's milk is a high fat fluid exquisitely designed to turn a 65 pound baby calf into a 400 pound cow. That's what cow's milk is for." The article also states that approximately half of the nation's entire antibiotics output goes into the feedstuff for animals and that "every sip of milk" can contain up to 59 different hormones.

I try to avoid all dairy products. If you continue to use them, I recommend that you do so in very limited amounts and that you eat raw, green, leafy vegetables along with them to aid in digestion and assimilation.

If you must have your milk, soy and rice milk are available

and taste great. And *don't* concern yourself about getting enough calcium. There are many other sources available. Broccoli, kale and other dark green vegetables along with soy, nuts and seeds are all great alternative sources of calcium.

My allergies disappeared for good when I eliminated dairy products from my life.

Refined and Processed Grains. Products made from bleached, processed flours like most breads, cakes, cereals, pastas and cookies, are extremely mucus and acid producing in the body.

Interesting Thought

Think of the paper mache projects you made in grade school. Remember the thick paste of flour and water? It also made a tough, hard glue when it dried. This is what is going into your body when you consume processed white flour products. Appetizing, isn't it?

Compared to fruits and vegetables, grains — even whole grains — can be lacking in important minerals. They are extremely acid forming in our bodies.

MUCUS PRODUCING FOODS

While this topic may be unpleasant to discuss, it is absolutely necessary if you are to bring health, vibrancy and energy into your life. Open your mouth and stick out your tongue. Give it a good look. Does it have a white coating? This is an indication of the mucus condition of your body. The more white you have on your tongue, the more mucus is in your system. Yes, I said mucus... thick and sticky mucus.

Because our human body and its complex systems are so incredible and efficient, we just expect it to keep rolling along no matter what we pump into it. Ron Langerquist and Tom McGregor state in their book, *The North American Diet*, that in America we pump over-processed, chemical laden, heavy, dairy rich foods into our bodies on a daily basis overloading our systems with this mucus. It clogs arteries, veins and organs just like cholesterol. When your body is overloaded with mucus, you can experience some very uncomfortable and unpleasant health issues such as colds, sore throats, fatigue, PMS symptoms, acne, boils and ear infections to name a few.

The function of mucus is to act as a lubricating agent which protects the mucus membranes along the digestive, respiratory, urinary and reproductive tracts. In its healthy state, this mucus is clear and slippery. Its functions also include stopping irritants, pollutants or carcinogenic compounds created by putrefying, undigested food residues. But as mucus and food move through the intestines, moisture is removed. When that happens, the mucus becomes increasingly sticky and thick and leaves a coating on the intestinal walls that builds up over time. This barrier can affect the ability to absorb nutrients. It is also an ideal environment for parasites to breed.

It is important to know that there are mucus *forming* and mucus *cleansing* foods. Certain foods cause an increase of mucus secretions. This substance is prone to putrefaction and can be toxic to the body. Its consistency is sticky and thick. When these particles are too large to pass through the membrane of a cell, they must remain in the colon until eliminated. If the body is overloaded with mucus and it is not cleansed from the systems, it can become stagnant and prone to infection.

Bread and milk cause sinus congestion in many people. They are not the only culprits. It is very important for us to realize what our way of eating is doing to us. We have the choice to change. Because you are reading this book, I believe you are in the process of making - or have already made - that choice. It will change your life completely. I have not had a cold, sore throat or the flu since starting this program and my allergies have completely disappeared. Make the choice to nurture your body instead of causing it harm.

Food Do's (Non-Mucus Forming)	Food Don'ts (Mucus Forming)
Vegetables	Refined Sugars
Fruits	Meat
Whole grains (sprouts)	Dairy Products
Nuts	Refined Flour Products
Seeds	Eggs
Fish (in small amounts)	Salt

In *The North American Diet*, the authors give a fine analogy of a system clogged with mucus; "Imagine a drain, clogged with human hair, dust, old soap and pieces of decaying food, all forming a sticky mass of rotting waste that cannot be removed. The medical names labeled for these diseases are diverticula, colitis, stricture, prolapsus, hemorrhoids, worm, yeast infection, chronic constipation, colon cancer and appendicitis." They go on to say, "Without the natural, sponge-like properties of fruits and vegetables, intestinal diseases will continue to abound, especially amongst the elderly." One of the most important steps I took in turning my life around was in eliminating virtually all mucus producing foods from my diet. That included meat, dairy products and most grain products including white breads, cereals, pastas, cakes and cookies. These are all highly acidic as well.

Up to the time I changed my eating patterns, I was consuming a great deal of cheese. I absolutely loved cheese of any kind, but especially the sharp cheddar variety. That, combined with a slice of sourdough bread, was a little piece of heaven to me. It had never occurred to me that the severe allergies which had plagued me for the previous 10 years or so might be somehow related to what I was eating. I would often have to sleep in a sitting position in order to breathe. Sinus headaches were also common at that time. I had been poked, prodded and scratched for every type of possible allergy, but the problems were never resolved. I had even resorted to allergy injections so that I could get some relief.

Then a funny thing happened. About three months after giving up dairy products, I found that the debilitating allergy symptoms I had been experiencing for so long were completely gone. I couldn't believe it. I could breathe easily out of both nostrils. I was able to sleep lying down. I no longer experienced sore throats, sinus headaches or heartburn. Virtually every symptom I had been suffering with was gone and *not one* has ever reappeared. I am allergy free and enjoy the wonderful feeling so much that I don't even miss the sharp cheddar!

Health Hints

- Grapes and citrus fruits are great mucus cleansers.
- Sufficient chewing and proper food combining also helps eliminate mucus congestion.

There are so many benefits to living on a mucus free program that it's hard to know where to start. Your body will be deeply cleansed. You will be full of energy and vitality. You will notice a definite decrease in body odors. You may not even need a deodorant. Puffiness and bloating will disappear. Your skin will look healthy, smooth and glowing. Fine facial lines will diminish or disappear. You will feel healthier. Your breath will be more pleasant. You will need less sleep and find it easier to focus your thinking. You will find that colds, flus and other ailments will pass you by.

WATER – THE OTHER LIQUID ASSET

Water, water everywhere… or at least that's the way it should be. If your goal is to keep your weight down and maintain a youthful beauty as you grow older, the importance of water cannot be overemphasized! Our bodies are made up of approximately 70% water. Look at a map of the earth. Look at the water on it. We have the same relationship of water in our bodies as the earth has. When you look at it from this angle, it is easy to see why water is so crucial to our health and our very life. Water plays an essential role in ALL aspects of body metabolism. Every function of the body is linked to the efficient flow of water. It has been said that the purest water in the world is the living water in raw plant foods. The only reason that people need to drink such large amounts of water (8-10 glasses per day) is because the foods they eat are massively dehydrated.

According to Alterra Healthcare Corporation, a leader in the assisted healthcare field, "On average, we drink only one cup of water each day. The rest of the water the body needs must be extracted from other liquids or foods we eat." This is crucial because, as they go on to state, "Small changes in the amount of water in your body can make a big difference." Each day the body loses substantial amounts of water through breathing, perspiration, and elimination.

They go on to add, "Even more water could be lost through exercise or hard work, excessively dry air, and alcohol and caffeine consumption. Stress, alcohol and caffeine all affect the amount of water and the speed in which your body loses it. Any of these factors alone or in combination could cause a small but critical shrinkage of the brain. This small shrinkage will impair neuromuscular coordination, decrease concentration, and slow thinking. Unfortunately, increased consumption of caffeine or alcohol is common in times of stress, resulting in loss of water."

Gary Null, Ph.D., recommends in his book *Ultimate Anti-aging Program* that we drink at least a gallon of purified water per day. He goes on to say that people get in the habit of drinking only at meal times or when noticeably thirsty. This decreases water consumed from the 74% water needed by your body to only 66-67%. He states that when your body doesn't have the amount of water it requires, you won't ever have the energy you need. "The very first thing I do to get people's energy up is to increase the amount of water in their diet. Immediately, their energy goes up. When someone has dementia, the first thing I do is give them lots of cold water all day, every day. About three weeks later, I start to see their dementia dissipate because they have rehydrated their brains. Unfortunately, your brain actually shrinks as you dehydrate. By drinking lots of pure water you get better neuron activity and better cellular chemistry and you're able to detoxify the cells with water."

I have found that I feel my best, fine facial lines minimize and I am more energetic when I consume 3 – 4 quarts (12 – 16 cups) of purified water every day. Even if I am consuming foods with a very high water content, I still feel better when I drink at least 3 quarts of water per day. I have learned to listen very closely to what my body tells me. It lets me know when I need more water and when I have had enough.

As I changed my lifestyle and started to make purified water my beverage of choice the symptoms of arthritis I had been experiencing began to disappear. Previously when I would play tennis, I would have to run warm water over my hands to "loosen up" the joints. But as I consumed more water, the pain I had been experiencing in my joints began to disappear. I now have no pain whatsoever in any of the joints of my body.

I also began to notice other benefits. The little pockets of cellulite that had begun to accumulate began to disappear. My thinking seemed to be clearer. Headaches have all but disappeared from my life. I can't tell you the last time I had to take an aspirin. In fact, if I begin to get a headache, I drink a couple of glasses of water and cut my consumption of food way down and within a short time the headache disappears. I had previously had problems with heartburn and ulcers. They have been completely eliminated. The fine lines on my face diminished and my complexion was clear and smooth. People began asking me what type of make-up I was using.

Then, of course, there is the "pleasant" subject of constipation. One of the main functions of the large intestines is to remove water from the waste. When a person is dehydrated the waste becomes hardened which makes its passage more difficult... leading to constipation. Therefore, more water equals less constipation.

I recommend a Warm Lemon-Water Flush first thing every morning. I have done this for years. It helps flush the kidneys, the liver and colon. It assists in the elimination of any waste from the digestive tract and bowels.

Warm Lemon-Water Flush

- 8 oz. warm, purified water
- Juice of 1/2 lemon
- Pinch of cayenne pepper (optional)

Combine all ingredients for a warm beverage to start your day.

The lemon juice helps to dislodge and flush the mucus that is clogged in the system. Lemon is a natural cleanser. It aids in liver detoxification.

The cayenne may be added for additional cleansing power. It stimulates digestive juices and helps eliminate the mucus.

From my own experience, I adamantly support the beneficial findings of adequate water consumption. I have concerns as to chemicals which are added to tap water, so I choose purified or distilled water whenever possible.

So little is known about the real benefits of adequate water consumption. I had an experience, not long ago, that magnifies my concern. I was browsing in a local bookstore and was beginning to feel thirsty. I approached the counter person at the franchise coffee concession and asked if they sold bottled water. We talked a moment as I was paying for my water and she wrinkled her nose and said to me, "Uchh… I can't believe people would choose to drink water when there are so many other good things to drink like coffee, cola and things like that!" This young woman had no idea what role water played in her ongoing health and well-being, not to mention her beauty.

Excessive weight gain and its relationship to adequate water consumption has been addressed in the book *Your Body's Many Cries for Water* written by F. Batmanghelidj: "We eat primarily to supply the brain with the energy needed for its round-the-clock work. The brain gets energy from two sources: either from sugar in blood circulation, or "hydroelectricity" produced as water is pumped through cell membranes. When the brain needs energy, it puts out signals of either thirst or hunger. Unfortunately, most people do not recognize these signals as thirst signals, only as hunger signals. Only about 20% of the food we eat reaches the brain. The rest goes to other parts of the body and will eventually become stored if muscle activity does not use it up. Since water moving through the cell membrane also can create energy for the brain, it is better to drink water instead of eating food. Excess does not store and create weight gain like excess food does. Therefore, drinking sufficient amounts of water helps reduce overeating."

So next time you reach out to grab a candy bar for a quick fix, try drinking a cool, soothing glass of water. I know it works… I have been doing this for years.

It should also be mentioned that water is especially important when the weather is very hot or very cold. It acts as a body temperature control. In the summer, perspiring helps keep body temperature within a normal range. In the winter, water acts as insulation.

Remember that caffeine is not just a stimulant, it is also a diuretic and will cause fluid loss. Therefore, only count *decaffeinated* drinks toward meeting your daily fluid requirements.

When we are speaking of water's contribution to beauty, it is important to remember that water carries away wastes and it hydrates the skin…both very important to the aspects of beauty and anti-aging of the skin. Drinking plenty of water also aids in releasing retained fluids. If your body does not have the water it needs, the body will hold on to the water it already has in an attempt to keep from losing it

So why should we care if water consumption is a major part of our lifestyle change? Because water:

- Suppresses the appetite.
- Assists the body in metabolizing stored fat.
- Reduces fat deposits in the body (cellulite loss).
- Relieves fluid retention problems.
- Hydrates and "plumps up" the skin.
- Reduces sodium buildup in the body.
- Helps maintain proper muscle tone.

- Rids the body of waste and toxins.
- Relieves constipation.
- Is a source of energy.

How much water should we consume in a day? Most experts agree that we should be drinking at least 64 ounces (2 quarts) of water per day and that we should drink an additional 8 ounces per day for every 25 pounds of excess weight. Some experts recommend that we drink cold water, since it is absorbed quicker and may burn more calories. I drink room temperature water since I feel it puts less strain on the system. Most importantly, always drink purified water.

I guarantee that once you start drinking two or more quarts of water per day, you will soon discover that you will not want to be without it. You will notice the visible differences when you are not providing yourself with the water your body needs. Treat your body lovingly. Provide it with what it needs and it will take care of you in wonderful ways!

Health Hint

A word about drinking liquids with meals. Try not to drink with your meals if possible. If you must, try to limit it to less than a cup of water. Liquids can make digestion much more difficult by diluting digestive juices. Cold drinks shut down digestive activity. I usually drink a couple of 16 oz. glasses of water about a half an hour to an hour before lunch or dinner and try to drink nothing with my meals. It helps to fill me and it doesn't interfere with digestion during my meals.

Eating foods with high water content is a great way to supply your body with the water it needs. As an added plus, these foods also supply essential nutrients. In his book *The Sunfood Diet Success System*, author David Wolfe provides a list of nutritious foods and their water content. Below is a short list to show you the differences in various fruits and vegetables. A full list is provided in the Appendix. You may want to refer to this list the next time you visit the market.

Food	Water Content
Fruit:	
Cucumbers	96%
Apples	84%
Avocados	75%
Olives (sun-ripened)	70%
Dates (fresh)	55%
Prunes (dried)	35%
Vegetables:	
Endive	94%
Lettuce	94%
Asparagus	93%
Bok Choy	87%
Kale	65%
Garlic Root	64%
Nuts & Seeds (unsoaked):	
Coconut water	92%
Coconut (young)	64%
Walnuts	25%
Sunflower Seeds	15%

As you can see, the water content of nuts is quite low due to their dense concentration. It is also important to remember that all green leafy vegetables are high water content and should be eaten liberally.

GREEN THINGS

"Several carefully studied populations in Mediterranean countries and in some areas in Asia where traditional diets consist largely of foods of plant origin exhibit long life expectancies and low rates of many chronic diseases. Studies provide further evidence that high consumption of vegetables confers numerous health benefits. The carotenoids as well as the vitamins, minerals, and fiber that are abundant in the plant-based diet appear to play impor-

tant roles in the prevention of several cancers, coronary heart disease, neural tube defects, and cataracts."
— Walter C. Willett, M.D., Dr. P.H.
Harvard School of Public Health

Green has become one of my favorite colors. It is the color of life. I try to eat as many green leafy vegetables as I can each day. The darker green, the better. Virtually all recommended vitamins and trace minerals are found in these colorful plants. They are full of life-giving water. These live green foods contain chlorophyll and are packed with living enzymes, which is so necessary to the assimilation of nutrients in our bodies. In plants, this chlorophyll is equivalent to blood in humans and animals. In fact, the only difference between human blood and chlorophyll is the center element in the chlorophyll molecule (magnesium). In human blood (hemoglobin), the center element of the molecule is iron. Chlorophyll is a natural blood builder. Even the oxygen we breathe comes from the chlorophyll in plants. Guess what… no chlorophyll, no life.

Yoshihide Hagiwara, M.D. in *Green Barley Essence* (Keats Publishing, 1985) states, "Plants are the 'lungs' of the planet, breathing out the oxygen all animal life needs to live. Plants are also the primary source of all that is of nutritional value."

Chlorophyll heals wounds and repairs damaged tissues. It inhibits the growth of bacteria and even controls halitosis (bad breath). It is an antioxidant that can actually be more effective than the Vitamin A, C or E antioxidants. In addition, it releases carbon dioxide from our bodies. Plants (green plant food sources) take carbon dioxide and carbon monoxide, the toxic by-products of our breathing and pollution, and turns them into usable oxygen for our systems.

Let's talk calcium and green foods. I constantly have people say to me, "How do you get your calcium if you don't eat dairy products?" They are always surprised to find out that green foods are far richer in calcium that can be easily absorbed in the body than milk. When I gave up dairy products and increased my intake of deep green leafy vegetables, my nails became stronger, my hair began to grow in more thickly and had shine to it. By the way, my last physical examination returned with an emphatic thumbs up on my bone density. It has also been reported that calcium can even reverse osteoporosis.

Leafy green vegetables are also body builders. They contain all the essential amino acids we require which make them a good source of protein. For those who believe that meat protein is essential for strength, it is interesting to note the world's strongest animals, such as the gorilla, hippopotamus, rhinoceros, elephant, zebra and giraffe, all build their powerful bodies with leafy greens.

Green foods provide a host of additional benefits to the body. They help clean the intestine of toxins. They provide essential fiber that assists in the elimination process of waste so that it doesn't sit in the intestine producing poisonous substances. Green foods contain potassium and cell salts that also aid in the proper elimination process of our systems. They are great tooth scrubbers and are powerful foods for healthy eyes.

As discussed previously, we know that our bodies require a pH of 7.35 to 7.45 to be considered in the healthy area. It has been reported that most Americans fall between 5 and 6 on the pH scale. No wonder there is so much acid indigestion around. However, by consuming dark green leafy vegetables we are helping to alkalize our systems while at the same time helping to flush out toxins.

Taking an antacid is not the answer. Antacids neutralize the digestive juices. Hence that hamburger, pizza, or steak and potato combination now sits in your stomach. It can't digest, because the digestive juices are neutralized, so it just sits there putrefying. Later, you eat a similar meal for dinner. The food from lunch is still sitting there, undigested. The new meal is dumped onto this and the whole mess just festers, creating poisons in your system. A disease-friendly environment begins to develop.

Disease is not inevitable. Negative body conditions can be reversed. Medical research is filled with miraculous stories. When we begin to take care of ourselves in a loving and natural way, our body responds in kind. Consuming living foods filled with working enzymes is vital to this process. The nutrient power found in dark green leafy vegetables is always more preferable to synthetic medicines and supplements since this is the way nature intended us to ingest these nutrients. And don't be fooled... your cells *do* know the difference!

One last wonderful bit of news: leafy green vegetables have virtually ZERO calories! All these benefits and no calories!

Along with the raw vegetables I eat each day, I try to consume at least 1 oz. of wheat grass juice or one 12-16 oz. glass of juiced vegetables including spinach, parsley, celery, beets and their greens, carrots, cucumbers, kale, wheat grass and spirulina. The Wild Oats Markets in my area make a juice drink called "The Earth Goddess" that incorporates all of these vegetables. I find that these drinks are real energizers as well as powerful nutrient providers. I realize that this may not be for everyone, but I have found such success with them that I have to speak their praise. If this is not for you, just add as many dark green vegetables to your meals as possible. Look around the produce section of your supermarket or health food store. You will find an abundance of variety of green foods. Try as many as you can. Mixed together, they make wonderful salads.

I personally prefer to consume my greens in a raw or live state. However, there are some very reliable concentrated products on the market. These can easily be mixed with juices or water. Check your nearest health food store to see what they offer. Below is a list of fine concentrated green products you might want to try:

1. Green Kamut Wheat Grass by Organic By Nature
   562-901-0177
   askgrassman@greenkamutcorp.com

2. Miracle Greens "TM"
   800-521-5867
   www.miracle-greens.com

3. Green Vibrance "R" – by Vibrant Health Division of TAAG Ltd.
   800-242-1835
   www.vibranthealth.org

4. ProGreens "R" by Nutricology
   800-545-9960
   www.nutricology.com

Health Hint

To wash non-organic fruits and vegetables, add 4 tablespoons salt and the juice of 1/2 lemon to a sink full of cold water. This makes a diluted form of hydrochloric acid. Soak for 2-3 minutes then rinse.

FABULOUS FRUIT

> *"Imagine the publicity if someone announced that they have developed a new treatment that cured 40 percent of all people with cancer. The media would be jumping up and down. That kind of benefit can be achieved to-day just by following a vegetarian diet. Right there you have an answer and no one's listening."*
> Oliver Alabaster, M.D.,
> Director of the Institute for Disease
> Prevention, George Washington
> University, Washington, D.C.

Nature has not only provided us a feast for our bodies, but a feast for our eyes when it comes to fruits and vegetables. Their beautiful colors span the rainbow. Nature has even used the intensity of color to give us clues as to express the intensity of nutrients and antioxidants within these powerful little packages. The more vibrant the color of the plant, the greater the nutrient content.

Fruits are Nature's natural body cleansers and detoxifiers. These wonderful, tasty little power packs are loaded with good stuff. First of all, they taste heavenly. Water makes up 80 to 95% of most fruits. Therefore, they are low in calories and provide you with essential internal moisture in its purest form. They are great sources of fiber which is essential in elimination of body waste and maintaining low cholesterol levels. Fruits are rich in both vitamins and minerals. Red, yellow and orange fruits are rich in carotenoids and flavonoids; blue, purple, and magenta are rich in anthocyanins; all of which function as serious antioxidants. Collagen, an intercellular substance that gives tissue its structure and keeps skin from wrinkling, is greatly enhanced by flavonoids.

Fruit contains a small quantity of protein, but it is of a high quality and is highly digestible. Fruits with higher protein content include apricots, avocados, bananas, cherries, dates, figs, and grapes.

Fruits generally fall into one of three categories: Sweet, Acid or Sub-acid. Sub-acid fruits are simply fruits that fall between sweet fruits and acid fruits in acidity and, therefore, can really be eaten with either type of fruit. They are slightly acidic.

There is an endless number of wonderful fruits to choose from. Who said that things have to taste bad to be good for you?

VERSATILE VEGETABLES

While fruits are Nature's natural cleansers, vegetables are Nature's natural body builders. Vegetables contain valuable antioxidants and protectants for the body. How much importance do you put on vegetables? When you sit down to eat, what takes up the most room on your plate? Your meat or vegetable serving? Most Americans consider vegetables to be a minor side dish to an oversized portion of meat of some kind.

Red, yellow, orange and purple vegetables, like their fruit counterparts, are loaded with anthocyanins, carotenoids and flavonoids with valuable antioxidant properties. They are also rich in vitamins C and E and fiber. This means they provide protection against disease and aging. Vegetables are also rich in vitamin A, folic acid, chlorophyll and other nutrients.

Were you aware that a salad can be a good source of protein? Most people aren't. The protein in green leaves is of extremely high quality. These leaves contain all essential amino acids plus a small quantity of essential fatty acids. The protein that the salad contains is not a large amount, but is highly digestible. It does not ferment in your intestines like other forms of protein can. In addition these green vegetables also contain alkaline minerals which help to assimilate protein.

Vegetables with good antioxidant properties are:

- Alfalfa sprouts
- Broccoli
- Cabbage
- Celery
- Eggplant
- Green beans
- Leaf Lettuce
- Potatoes
- Spinach
- Sweet Potatoes
- Yellow squash
- Beets
- Brussels sprouts
- Carrots
- Cucumbers
- Garlic
- Kale
- Onions
- Red Peppers
- Sweet corn
- Tomatoes

Again, let the colors be your guide. Look for the darkest, richest, most vibrant colors when picking out your vegetables.

Wheat Grass

Wheat grass is considered by many to be Nature's finest medicine. It has been referred to as a "green sunlight transfusion."

One ounce of wheat grass provides the equivalent in vitamins, minerals and amino acids of 2 – 2 1/2 pounds of green leafy vegetables. The nutrients from this juice are completely assimilated by the human body in 20 minutes. This is a source of quick energy. It also contains antioxidant properties. It is packed full of chlorophyll, active enzymes, vitamins and other nutrients. This emerald colored juice is one of the richest natural sources of vitamins A, complete B complex, B-17, C, E and K. It also provides an excellent source for Calcium, Potassium, Iron, Magnesium, Phosphorus, Sodium, Sulfur, Cobalt, Zinc, 17 forms of amino acids and enzymes. Chlorophyll makes up over 70% of the solid content of wheat grass juice. Wheat grass is a great aid in weight loss. It is known to suppress appetite, stimulate metabolism and circulation and increase energy.

Wheat grass has been linked to numerous additional benefits:

- Rebuilds blood.
- Builds immune properties.

- Helps prevent tooth decay.
- Improves the body's ability to heal.
- Neutralizes carcinogens in the body.
- Eliminates toxins and cleanses the body.
- The chlorophyll is an internal deodorant.
- Reduces high blood pressure.
- Helps purify the liver.
- Improves digestion.
- Improves blood sugar disorders.
- Keeps hair from graying.
- Removes heavy metals from the body.

This wonderful green juice is an essential part of my diet now. Wheat grass juice has a sweet, earthy flavor. Some authorities recommend up to 4 ounces per day for optimal health. While I do not take issue with that, I find that an ounce a day supplies me with the benefits and energy I desire.

Start with 1 oz. per day and work your way up to what feels right for you. Wheat grass can be a bit overpowering if you take larger doses when you are just beginning to consume the juice.

I enjoy drinking my wheat grass straight. However, most health food stores that have a juice bar will have numerous vegetable and fruit drinks that can be added to your wheat grass if you prefer. I often blend my own drinks at home. If you choose to go this route, you will need to purchase a juicer. It extracts the pulp while leaving you a rich, nutrient packed drink. Wheat grass requires a special juicer for extracting the juice from the fine blades of grass or you can purchase wheat grass juice at a health food store.

My favorite drink is a mixture of:
- Beets
- Carrots
- Cucumber
- Kale
- Parsley
- Spinach
- Wheat grass

The color is nothing to write home about but the energy kick will keep you going all day. There are more vegetable nutrients packed in one of these drinks than most people consume in one week. I always have my drinks stirred, not blended, since nutrients are lost through the oxygenation process that occurs during blending.

Two more wheat grass combinations to try:
Carrot – Wheat grass Juice Drink
- 1 oz. Wheat grass juice
- 3 oz. Carrot juice

Pineapple – Wheat grass Juice Drink
- 1 oz. Wheat grass juice
- 1 oz. Pineapple juice

Wheat grass can also be used externally as:
- a scalp treatment for lusterous hair
- a cleanser/astringent for all types of skin
- a treatment for blocked sinuses
- a stimulant for circulation (rub into skin)
- a treatment to help heal cuts and bruises more quickly

SEA GREENS
Spirulina
This is a form of blue green sea algae that gets its name from its corkscrew shape. The United Nations has proclaimed, "Spirulina is the most ideal food for mankind." The U.S. Department of Agriculture in 1988 published "Spirulina: Food For the Future." It is the earth's oldest living plant and is the most nutritionally concentrated food known to man.

The iron in this mega food is 58 times richer that that of raw spinach and easier to digest. Spirulina is composed of about 65% protein. The protein in spirulina is twice that of soybeans and at least three times that of beef, fish or eggs. The amino acids in spirulina are in a form that is perfect for instantaneous assimilation.

Additional benefits of Spirulina:

- Stimulates immune system to destroy invading disease organisms and carcinogens
- Detoxifies the colon
- Promotes tissue repair
- Has anti-infectious properties
- Decreases cholesterol levels
- Works as an anti-inflammatory
- Helps balance RNA and DNA
- Curbs appetite
- Helps stimulate metabolism

Generally only small amounts of this powerful food needs to be consumed to receive great benefits.

Sea Vegetables

Seaweeds, or sea vegetables, are extremely rich in vitamins, minerals and nutrients. They are also extremely high in calcium and phosphorous. Approximately 25% of seaweed is protein and only about 2% is fat. These little vegetables are also low in calories.

Besides containing virtually all of the minerals and vitamins that are useful in preventing free radical formation, sea vegetables are known for their effect on dissolving fat deposits and eliminating heavy metal contaminants from the body. They have also been used in lowering blood cholesterol, thinning the blood and even cancer treatment.

Sea vegetables are an amazing food source.

The next time you are at your favorite Japanese restaurant, try ordering a seaweed salad. You may think it sounds strange, but don't let that stop you. The first time I ordered it I was apprehensive too. Now it is one of my favorites. It is served topped with tofu squares and tossed with a wonderful sesame dressing. It's delicious!

Health Hint

Soak seaweed for at least 1/2 hour before preparation. This will reduce the sodium content.

Kelp

Kelp is actually a form of seaweed. It is usually dried or ground into power but can be eaten raw. Tablets are available for those who don't like the taste.

Kelp provides a number of nutritional benefits:

- A very good source of vitamins, minerals and trace elements
- Good for nails
- Good for brain tissue and membranes surrounding the brain
- Good for blood vessels and sensory nerves
- Useful in the treatment of thyroid problems
- Used in the treatment of hair loss
- Used in the treatment of obesity

I have found that when I am consuming kelp, my skin feels much softer. I take about 1 teaspoon per day mixed in juice or water.

FATS AND OILS/ESSENTIAL FATTY ACIDS

As I sat watching the evening news a short time ago, I found myself stunned by what I was hearing. Here was a woman being interviewed who stated she had dieted her whole life but each time resulted in dismal failure. So she had decided to follow the latest fad diet, one which she stated was contrary to everything she had believed up to that point. She had begun eating a diet which consisted primarily of fat. She did not appear to have any understanding of the difference between *good* fat and *bad* fat. Just as long as it was fat, that is all that mattered. This appeared to be a well educated, intelligent woman. Yet in her desperation, she was forging forward on what could be a catastrophic journey.

It's as if we have been willing to try anything and everything, except what will actually work. Everything in existence adheres to one or more of Nature's Laws. There is no getting around it. There is no cheating. You may lose weight temporarily on some fad diet, but when you are not following the fundamental laws of eating, you will soon put the weight back on. Depending how radical the diet has been, you may cause irreparable damage to the body. You can't cheat the Laws of Nature. When you eat in a manner that aligns with Nature, your body will respond with thanks by fulfilling your desire: shedding the burdensome excess weight and providing you with glowing health and energy beyond your wildest expectations.

Essential fatty acids are just that — essential! These fatty acids are necessary for the health of the cells but the body cannot manufacture them itself. These acids provide a number of functions such as healing, carrying vitamins, stimulating skin and hair growth, enhancing metabolism and bringing oxygen to the tissues. They can act as a solvent to remove hardened fat. They can even help you lose weight. They have been shown to play a preventive role in the skin aging process. Always purchase *cold pressed* oils since heat, light, air and commercial processing can destroy their effectiveness.

Polyunsaturated Fats

The two Polyunsaturated Fats (PUFAs) that cannot be made by the body include:

- *Alpha-Linoleic acid (ALA) – (Omega 3)*
  Found in hemp seed, flax seed, pumpkin seed, walnuts, dark green leaves, canola, soybean, spirulina and cold water fish.
- *Linoleic Acid (LNA) – (Omega 6)*
  Found in safflower, hemp seed, soybean, walnuts, pumpkin seed, sesame seed, corn, avocado, evening primrose, sunflower and flax seed.

Health Hint

Adding oils to your daily diet will help you get the essential fatty acids that your body needs. It is important that these oils be added in an *unheated* form.

Flax Seed Oil – an internal Beauty Cream.

Add 2 tablespoons of cold pressed Flax oil to your daily diet. Flax is one of the best sources of Omega 3 oils. It can reverse the degenerative process and provides moisture and necessary oils from the inside. I noticed that after taking flax oil consistently for about a month, my skin was much softer and fine facial lines disappeared. I highly recommend a dose-a-day.

Olive Oil

Add 1 tablespoon of cold pressed Extra Virgin Olive oil (Omega 9) to your daily diet. Olive oil appears to protect against heart disease and the prevention of cancer. Be sure that you only buy *Extra Virgin*, not *Pure*. Pure is a mixture and is a refined product.

Saturated Fats

Saturated fats are called saturated because the carbon atoms of the molecular structure are saturated with hydrogen atoms. These saturated fats come in both the good and bad variety. An example of *good* saturated fat is found in avocados and olives. These fats are easy to digest and are nutritious. Raw nuts are another good example, however they are more difficult to digest. These foods have been unaffected by light, air or heat.

The body protects itself against starvation by storing fat, but it doesn't particularly care what kind of fat it stores. Meat, white sugar, refined flours and dairy products are stored as thick, sticky fat that can increase the risk of stroke, heart attack and arteriosclerosis.

In the July 12, 2002 issue of *Freedom: Your Nutrition Center* newsletter, the following incident is cited: "Dr. Klapper had a patient who was scheduled for by-pass surgery in the morning. When he drew the blood for analysis, floating in the test tube was a thick, greasy, white, sticky film. When the patient was asked what he had had for lunch, he replied, 'A cheeseburger and milk shake.' The surgeon realized that what he had seen in the test tube was the fat from his patient's lunch. During the operation on the following day, Dr. Klapper pulled a 4-inch long yellow sausage of fatty material from the man's artery which was depriving the heart of oxygen." The article goes on to provide the amazing statistic that seventy-five percent of North Americans die due to diseases related to fat consumption. (I wonder how many people following the fat consumption diet have read this statistic.)

While we don't tend to think of white sugar and starches in terms of fat, it is a valid concern to look at. White sugar, white flour, white rice, pasta, corn starch, tapioca and most breakfast cereals convert to saturated fat. These foods overload the blood with glucose and the body then turns the excess into *body fat*.

Saturated fats from animal sources and vegetable oils tend to stick together and form hard plaques in the arteries. These saturated fats from animal sources are common culprits in the development of fatty, degenerative disease.

- *Monounsaturated oils.* Monounsaturated fatty acids such as olive and canola oil have a different molecular structure from saturated fatty acid molecules which renders them more fluid. Olive oil appears to play a beneficial role in prevention of heart disease.

- *Polyunsaturated oils.* Polyunsaturated fatty acid molecules are even more fluid and more likely to spoil easily. Safflower and corn oil are examples.

- *Synthetic Trans Fats.* These are killer fats — plain and simple. Try to eliminate margarine, shortening, deep fried foods cooked in hydrogenated high-heated oil, processed animal products and any packaged foods such as chips, cookies, bread, etc., which have partially hydrogenated fat listed on the packaging. A consistent diet of these foods promotes aging and degenerative disease.

    In their book *Over 50 Looking 30!* Nina Anderson and Howard Peiper state, "One very important reason for men to avoid trans-fats and balance EFAs (Essential Fatty Acids) is that baldness may be avoided. A report on the correlation between heart attacks and baldness reveals that the gunk created by trans-fats adheres to both the arterial wall and hair follicles. This plaque builds up smothering the hair and preventing it from getting oxygen. Thus hair actually stops growing because it is buried under layers of fatty goo. Once these layers are cleaned off and the trans-fats eliminated from the diet, dormant hair may actually emerge intact, or new growth will be regenerated."

- *Cholesterol.* Without cholesterol hormones such as estrogen, progesterone, and testosterone would not be made. Cholesterol helps prevent dehydration and contributes to the skin's healing process and may act as an antioxidant.

  However, the more animal proteins you eat, the higher the level of cholesterol that accumulates. High levels of cholesterol cause hardening of the arteries. This cholesterol is hard, waxy and very resistant to breakdown in the body.

  According to writer, John Henkel, in his article "Keeping Cholesterol Under Control" in the January-February, 1999 internet issue of *FDA Consumer Magazine*, "Low-density lipoprotein (LDL) — this "bad" cholesterol is the form in which cholesterol is carried into the blood and is the main cause of harmful fatty buildup in arteries. The higher the LDL cholesterol level in the blood, the greater the heart disease risk." He goes on to state, "High-density lipoprotein (HDL) helps prevent a cholesterol buildup in blood vessels. Low HDL levels increase heart disease risk." He also states, "Menopause is often associated with increases in LDL cholesterol in women."

It should be noted that while animal proteins and fats *raise* serum cholesterol levels, fruits, vegetables, nuts, seeds and beans cause cholesterol levels to *fall*.

Fats To Avoid	
Beef	Liver
Butter	Margarine
Cheese	Whole Milk
Egg Yolk	

Including natural fat sources such as avocados, olives, nuts, seeds, raw coconut, flax and olive oils to your diet will aid you immensely in transitioning from a cooked food diet to a raw plant-based diet. These foods take longer to digest and keep the body feeling fuller for a longer period of time. This prevents your body from experiencing dips in energy. These natural plant fat sources also serve as internal lubricants and beauty creams for the skin, hair and body joints.

Nuts & Seeds

The controversy goes on concerning nuts. Is their consumption helpful or harmful? In general, nuts are very nutritious. They provide protein and important vitamins such as A and E. They contain phosphorous, potassium and fiber. However, they are high in fat and most nuts are also acid producing (almonds and Brazil nuts tend to be less acid). Just limit the amount of nuts you consume.

Be sure to keep nuts in a cool, dry area away from light. Keeping them in an airtight container in the refrigerator will help keep them from turning rancid.

Soaking the nuts in water from 2 hours to overnight will aid in their digestibility. This will rehydrate them, activating their enzymes and makes them more easily digestible. Be sure to eat raw nuts and leave the salted and roasted variety alone.

Pumpkin or sunflower seeds make delicious, crunchy and nutrient packed additions to your salads. By combining them with dark leafy greens, the body can more easily digest them.

PROTEIN

Proteins are the building blocks of life and provide us with energy. Our diets must contain them. However, research shows that Americans eat up to five times the amount of protein their body actually needs. When asked where they get protein from in their diet, most people will respond that their protein comes from meat. Eating too much protein from meat puts the body in a highly acidic state.

Proteins are made from amino acids. There are 22 amino acids found in the body, 14 of which the body is capable of producing on its own. The remaining 8 essential amino acids can ALL be found in abundance in raw plant foods like green leafy vegetables. Strict food combining is not necessary to get adequate protein. Protein supplements are unnecessary, expensive and may actually be harmful to some individuals.

Concerns about not getting enough protein in your diet is unfounded. Alkaline foods, such as fruits and vegetables con-

97

tain protein, promote health and aid in weight loss. When choosing your protein, choose quality protein sources that have not been pumped full of hormones, pesticides and other toxins. Digesting protein can take approximately two to six hours depending on the type of protein you eat. This keeps you feeling full for longer periods of time.

The RDA (Recommended Daily Allowance) for protein is about 0.36 grams of protein for each pound that you weigh. Rid yourself of the fear of not getting enough protein. Rid yourself of the misconception that you must get your protein from animal products. Good choices would be:

- Almonds
- Avocados
- Beans
- Green Leafy Vegetables
- Mushrooms (in moderation)
- Nuts
- Soy Milk
- Soy Nuts
- Sprouted Grains & Legumes
- Sunflower seeds
- Tempeh
- Tofu

CALCIUM

Many people ask me, "How do you get enough calcium if you are not consuming dairy products?" They worry that a calcium deficiency will develop if milk products are eliminated from their diet.

All leafy green vegetables and grasses are high in calcium. (How do you think cows get their calcium?) Celery, kale, broccoli, dried fruit, cauliflower, okra, onions, green beans, avocado, black beans, garbanzo beans (chickpeas), tofu, almonds, hazelnuts and sesame seeds are other good sources of calcium.

One of calcium's jobs is to neutralize the body when you have consumed acid forming foods like animal protein and dairy products. If there is not enough calcium on hand, the body will take it from the cells of your body, for example, the cells in your bones. There are nutritional experts who feel that a lack of calcium is not the problem concerning osteoporosis, but that the over-consumption of animal protein and dairy products is the culprit. As mentioned earlier, salt also depletes calcium. A list of alkalizing foods and their calcium content can be found in the Appendix.

VITAMINS AND MINERALS – THE QUESTION OF SUPPLEMENTS

"Let food be your medicine and your medicine be your food."

– Hippocrates
Father of Western Medicine

It has been reported that about half of the people in this country take at least one supplement on a regular basis. Many take handfuls per day. You know the old thought process that goes, "if one is good, then a whole handful must be great!" In the case of supplements, this just may not be so. While vitamins and minerals are necessary to the healthy functioning of the body's enzymes, too much of certain supplements can actually have a harmful effect on your body. Vitamins do not, in themselves, provide usable energy for the body. The job of vitamins is to help the body's enzymes to release energy from the carbohydrates, proteins and fats that are ingested. Minerals are organic elements that are absolutely essential for the proper functioning of the body.

There are two types of vitamins: water-soluble and fat-soluble.

- *Water soluble.* These vitamins dissolve in water. They are absorbed into the blood stream and then into the cells as needed. These are usually safe even in higher amounts because any excess is expelled fairly readily by the system. Vitamins B Complex and C are water soluble vitamins.

- *Fat soluble.* These vitamins do not dissolve in the blood stream. Because of this they can accumulate in the body resulting in toxic amounts. The fat soluble vitamins are vitamins A, D, E and K.

Vitamins help regulate metabolism. Vitamins A, C and E are also known as antioxidants. These vitamins fight the harmful effects of free radicals roaming our bodies. They interfere with the proper functioning of free radicals… and that is a good thing.

Unfortunately, many people take vitamins as a shortcut to

good health. They continue to eat the same dead foods, but feel that ingesting supplements will provide them with the necessary nutrients they need to stay healthy. No real effort is made to change the lifestyle.

If you decide to add supplements to your diet, read the labels. Be aware that some companies add fillers or binders to the vitamins. Not all these fillers or binders are good for you. Be aware of time-released capsules. These capsules can be made of hydrogenated oils — this is what allows them to provide the slow release.

Be aware that there are *synthetic* vitamins and *natural* vitamins. Natural vitamins are obtained from food sources whereas synthetic vitamins are developed in laboratories. Synthetic vitamins are generally less expensive and have an extended shelf life. They do not contain the nutrients that vitamins derived from natural foods may have. More information regarding vitamins, minerals and their food sources are contained in the Appendix.

Remember — there is no replacement for the nutrition provided by the Greatest Diet on Earth — Nature's fresh foods.

MAKING YOUR FOOD WORK FOR YOU

Have you ever experienced indigestion, bloating, a burning sensation, headache and/or fatigue after eating a "hardy" meal? Of course, we all have. Most people, however, attribute these discomforts to overeating. While that may be the case in some instances, improper food combinations could be the culprit in the majority of cases. As we get older, our digestive tract works less efficiently. Digestion can take longer. We require fewer calories. Therefore it becomes increasingly important that we understand the elements of proper food combining to get the very most out of what we are putting into our bodies. We can no longer afford to mindlessly throw just any type of food into our system and expect to get optimal nutritional benefits from it. It is time for us to take responsibility for our health.

One of the most commonly overlooked aspects, yet one of the key elements of weight loss and energy gain, is the combining of our foods at meals. I noticed an immediate improvement in how I felt when I began applying the laws of proper food combining. When our meals are *simple* and *combined correctly*, our metabolism can work more rapidly and efficiently. Proteins require usually two to six hours to digest due to their high concentration. Carbohydrates run a close second in digestion time, usually two to four hours, due also to their concentration. Fruits are the least concentrated and will digest usually in an hour. Fats are digested very slowly. When fats are eaten with proteins, digestion is slowed almost to the point of stopping.

Our human digestive system is amazing. It is capable of digesting an astonishing array of foods. The key to remember is that the body was not meant to digest all these different foods at the same time. Different foods require different digestive enzymes. When these different digestive juices are all released into the system at the same time, they can bring digestion to a halt. Bloating, fermentation, gas, indigestion and toxin build-up begins to occur. When food is not properly digested it is not completely broken down in the body and it will not pass through the intestinal tract as it should. Undigested particles get stuck in pockets in the intestine. This undigested food becomes nourishment for damaging bacteria to feed upon.

The digestion of protein calls for a highly acidic environment whereas the digestion of starch, vegetables and fats call for a mildly alkaline environment. Basic chemistry laws remind us that acids and bases neutralize each other. Going back to the food that is sitting in your stomach, it sits there and ferments and then becomes a breeding ground for bacteria to decompose it. The by-products of this fermentation are toxic to your body.

It is important to remember that it is not just about eating healthy food. It's about eating combinations of healthy foods that allow your body to digest, utilize and assimilate the nutrients you are putting into it while eliminating the nonusable material as quickly as possible.

The simpler the meal, the less load on the digestive system. For example, lots of leafy green vegetables with a protein or starch food puts less strain on the digestive system, nutrients are assimilated properly and waste products can move through our system and be eliminated quickly. This leaves our bloodstream in a much purer state and more able to perform its functions.

For those of you who think antacids are the answer to indigestion, its time to take another look. Let's say you are experiencing major discomfort after a big meal of steak, baked potato topped with butter or margarine and sour cream with pie ala mode for dessert. So you pop an antacid and all is well. Right? Well, let's see. The antacid actually neutralizes the digestion of the foods in your system. The foods then sit there fermenting and putrefying. In fact, they will probably sit there until you eat your next typical American meal of processed foods and/or poor food combinations. This new food is dumped on an already fermenting, undigested mess and your system only becomes more uncomfortable. The answer is not the ingestion of pharmaceutical products, it is in the knowledge of properly combining foods. When your body is experiencing bloating, a burning sensation, indigestion, and/or a headache, *it is trying to tell you something!* Listen to it. It will always tell you what is right and wrong for your body. We need simply to listen.

Limitless delicious meals can be made with proper food combining. There are several good books out on this subject should you decide to study this further.

Making Your Food Work for You – Fundamental Laws
1. First and most important of all, don't tax the body by overeating any food. And chew your food very, very thoroughly.
2. Don't eat too many types of foods at the same meal.
3. Bread is easier to digest and is less mucus forming when lightly toasted. (Try to eat low sodium, sprouted grain bread...it makes terrific toast and digests very easily).
4. The major part of your diet should be vegetables and fruits. (Eat as many non-starchy vegetables as you desire.)
5. When eating foods containing protein, carbohydrates or fat, eat a leafy green salad. It aids in the digestion process.
6. Eat proteins and starches at different meals. Example: don't each a steak and baked potato at the same meal. The digestive juices will neutralize each other.

7. Eat only one kind of protein at any given meal.
8. Eat proteins and fats at separate meals. Nuts take hours to digest due to their extremely high fat content.
9. Eat proteins and sugars at separate meals.
10. Eat fruits alone if possible. Fruits should be eaten at least 15 minutes before a meal since they are held up during digestion when eaten in combination with other foods that require digestion in the stomach. This leads to fermentation.
11. Eat melons alone or leave them alone. These do not combine well with other foods.
12. Do not eat fruit or sweet, sugary concoctions for dessert. They lay on top of already ingested food in the stomach and ferment. The only fruit recommended for dessert is Papaya. The enzymes in the fruit actually aid in digestion.

The following charts will help you in your selection of foods to both alleviate indigestion problems and provide you with the maximum energy, weight loss and health benefits.

Examples of Foods that Work Most Effectively Together

Proteins and Non-Starches
Combine any food in the protein column with
any food in the vegetable column

Proteins	Green Leafy, Non-Starchy Vegetables	
Avocados	Artichokes	Mushrooms
Lentils	Asparagus	Okra
Nuts	Broccoli	Parsley
Olives	Cabbage	Peas
Seeds	Cauliflower	Peppers
Soybeans	Celery	Radishes
	Corn	Spinach
	Cucumbers	Sprouts
	Eggplant	Summer Squash
	Green Beans	(Yellow/Zucchini)
	Lettuce	Turnips

Starches and Non-Starches
Combine any food in the starches column with
any food in the vegetable column

Starches	Green Leafy, Non-Starchy Vegetables	
Beets	Artichokes	Okra
Carrots	Asparagus	Parsley
Corn (Dried)	Broccoli	Peas
Grains	Cabbage	Peppers
Legumes	Cauliflower	Radishes
Potatoes	Celery	Spinach
Pumpkins	Corn	Sprouts
Wild Rice	Cucumbers	Summer Squash
Winter Squash	Eggplant	(Yellow/Zucchini)
(Hubbard, Acorn,	Green Beans	Turnips
Butternut)	Lettuce	
	Mushrooms	

Fruits – Acid and Sub-Acid
Combine any food in the acid column with
any food in the sub-acid column

Acid Fruits	Sub-Acid Fruits	
Citrus Fruits (All)	All Core Fruits	Sweet Plums &
Cranberries	All Stone and Pit Fruits	Sweet Apples
Currants	Apricots	
Gooseberries	Blueberries, Raspberries	
Pineapples	Fresh Figs	
Pomegranates	Grapes	
Sour Apples	Mangoes	
Sour Cherries	Papaya	
Strawberries	Pears & Sweet Peaches	
Tomatoes	Sweet Cherries	

*Because Sub-Acid Fruits are neither sweet nor acid, they can be eaten
with either sweet or acid fruits.

Fruits – Sweet and Sub-Acid
Combine any food in the sweet column with
any food in the sub-acid column

Sweet Fruits	Sub-Acid Fruits	
Bananas	All Core Fruits	Mangoes
Dates	All Stone and Pit Fruits	Papaya
Dried Fruit (All)	Apricots	Pears & Sweet Peaches
Persimmons	Blueberries, Raspberries	Sweet Cherries
Sweet Grapes (All)	Fresh Figs	Sweet Plums &
	Grapes	Sweet Apples

*Because Sub-Acid Fruits are neither sweet or acid, they can be eaten with either sweet fruits or acid fruits.

Examples of Foods that Work Less Effectively Together

Fruits
Combining foods in the sweet column with
foods in the acid calcium is not recommended.

Sweet Fruits	Acid Fruits	
Bananas	Citrus Fruits (All)	Pomegranates
Dates	Cranberries	Sour Apples
Dried Fruit (All)	Currants	Sour Cherries
Persimmons	Gooseberries	Strawberries
Sweet Grapes (All)	Pineapples	Tomatoes

Proteins and Starches
Combining foods in the protein column with
foods in the starches column is not recommended.

Proteins	Starches	
Avocados	Beets	Pumpkins
Lentils	Carrots	Wild Rice
Nuts (All)	Corn (Dried)	Winter Squash
Olives	Grains (All)	(Hubbard, Acorn,
Seeds (All)	Legumes	Butternut)
Soybeans	Potatoes	

SPECIAL NOTES

Melons
Do not combine with other foods

Cantaloupes   Honey Dew Melons
Casaba Melons   Watermelons
Crenshaw Melons

Avocado
Actually a fruit. Since it is high in protein and low in sugar you can combine it with any vegetables and with grains. So enjoy that avocado, sprout and tomato sandwich on whole grain bread.

Tomato
Also a fruit. Raw tomatoes are acidic fruits, but they have an alkaline effect on the body because of its low sugar content. Tomatoes can be combined with any vegetable.

Lemons & Limes
Lemons and limes are acidic fruits, but they actually have an alkaline effect on the body. They can therefore be combined with starches, proteins or oils.

INTERESTING FACT
Vegetables and fruits have been shown to decrease the amount of calcium excreted in the urine. They do this by neutralizing the acids produced by meat and fish when the body digests them. These acids would normally increase the amount of calcium lost in the urine.

THE HEALTH BANDITS

Sugar – Let's Not Sugar Coat It
When the phrase "name your poison" was coined, refined sugar could have easily been the subject. As a toxin it's a superstar. Its calories are empty and non-nutritious. It clogs the system. Because sugars can ferment in your body, it can trigger a sour stomach.

Our body, cells and brain do, in fact, use simple sugar - or glucose — as fuel. Our liver and muscle tissues store this simple sugar as glycogen for future use. Our body stores any excess sugar as fat as a type of insurance in the event of starvation. This is a normal and natural function. However, for most people sugar consumption has all but become an addiction.

Part of the problem is how we view sweets. We show affection or reward behavior with sweet treats. As Elson M. Haas, M.D. states in his book, *The Detox Diet*, "Holidays and special occasions are centered around sugar — birthday cakes and ice cream, Halloween candy, chocolate Easter eggs, Thanksgiving pie, Christmas cookies, Valentine chocolates — the list is endless. Sweet talk is embedded in our language, sweetie, sweetie pie, sweetheart, honey, sugar, sugar baby, candy, sweet cakes, baby cakes, honey bun, sugar plum. The message is loud and clear: sweetness = love."

When a person overwhelms his or her system with sugar, hypoglycemia, a condition characterized by the body's inability to properly metabolize sugar, then can develop. Fatigue, dizziness, headaches, restlessness and confusion can all be symptoms of overconsumption of sugar. Even emotional and psychological problems like depression and anxiety have been linked to the consumption of sugar. In Dr. Elson Haas' book, *The Detox Diet*, he states that Emanuel Cheraskin, M.D., showed in 1976 that a single intake of sugar can lower the bacteria fighting capabilities of white blood cells in the blood for up to five hours in test subjects.

Blood sugar levels in the body can fluctuate wildly when excess sugar is consumed. When we are feeling tired and we eat a quick candy bar or sugar sweet as a quick fix, the sugar is absorbed extremely quickly. The pancreas can overreact and cause the blood sugar to take a rapid drop. We then experience mood swings, depression and a loss of energy.

The over consumption of sugar has been linked to many health problems including, but not limited to: cancer of the colon, rectum, breast, ovary, prostate, kidney, nervous system, pancreas, coronary artery disease, diabetes, digestive problems, hypoglycemia, dental cavities and premenstrual problems.

We need to be very aware of the labeling that we find on our food products. Sometimes it is very creative. If a label says "sugar free — sweetened with fructose," don't be fooled. Fructose, glucose, sucrose, maltose, lactose, dextrose, galactose and corn syrup are all forms of sugar. Sometimes a label may list several of these plus sugar. When you add them all up, it makes up an overwhelming percentage of the food product. According to Gary Null in his book, *Ultimate Lifetime Diet*, the average person eats up to 33 tablespoons of sugar a day! That's right... if you're like me you will have to read that statement again to believe it. One can of cola may contain 9 to 11 tablespoons of sugar and one cup of sweetened cereal may contain up to 7 tablespoons of sugar. It does not take much to make 33 tablespoons per day. *That adds up to 150 pounds of sugar consumed **each year** by the average person!* Sugar is an addictive substance, just like alcohol. Withdrawal symptoms such as headaches, chills and body aches are common.

Sugar is also an intoxicating substance which negatively affects neurotransmitters in the brain creating emotional disorders such as irritability, manic-depressive tendencies, difficulty concentrating, inconsistency in thoughts and actions, situational personality changes, emotional outbursts and eating disorders. Most of the sugar consumed by the average individual is in manufactured foods.

Be especially aware of products that are marketed as "low fat" or "all natural." What the manufacturer fails to mention is that these products are often the worst for added sugar because, for flavor purposes, when some of the fat is taken out of the product, sugar is often added.

Research has also shown that high calorie consumption causes our bodies to age more quickly. When we consume these empty calories from sugar, energy utilization is increased, which stresses and ages the body at a more rapid rate than normal.

I had frequent headaches prior to changing my food lifestyle. I also suffered mood swings that I could not account for. When I eliminated sugar, the headaches I had experienced were also eliminated from my life. The mood swings, anxiety and depression leveled out.

Fruits are so naturally sweet that they are an easy replacement for candy. Once sugar is eliminated, you will be more than pleasantly surprised to find that the juicy, light sweetness of a piece of fruit far surpasses the dry, heavy sweetness of refined sugar. There is a world of difference between the types of sweetness. Although I prefer fresh fruit to dried fruit, there are wonderful dried fruits such as papaya, pineapple and dates, which are extremely sweet and are excellent substitutes for refined sugar when that "sweet tooth" is calling. (Be sure your dried fruit is sulfur free.) Once you have made the switch, however, your taste buds become more sensitive to taste and the sweetness of refined sugar is less than appealing. On occasion, I have succumbed to the temptation of a donut loaded with sugar or a piece of chocolate cake at a party. But I have found that within about half an hour I notice the beginning of a headache.

When you eliminate sugar from your diet, you will notice that foods actually start to taste better. Your taste buds will become more sensitive to the real flavor and sweetness of foods. You will start to feel calmer, your thoughts will be clearer and you will lose your craving for overwhelmingly sweet foods. You will find that munching on a piece of fruit will satisfy your sweet cravings. Fruit won't trigger that overwhelming craving that white refined sugar does and allows you to stay in control and still enjoy a sweet treat. Keep in mind that even fruits are sources of sugar. I find that even dried fruit is now too sweet for me. A simple fresh mango, ripe banana, a bowl of fresh pineapple slices or one of my cantaloupe shakes totally satisfies my sweet tooth with the added benefit of cleansing toxins from and providing essential nutrients to my body. I can completely enjoy this snack and also know that it will have absolutely no negative effect on my weight or health.

Shocking Health Fact

Studies have shown that a single intake of sugar can lower the bacteria fighting capabilities and, in essence, shut down the immune system for up to 5 hours!

Aspartame – By Any Other Name

No discussion on sugar would be complete without mentioning the "other" sugar. Aspartame is the technical name for a sugar substitute known under the brand names of NutraSweet® and Equal®. In her article "Facts They Don't Want You To Know About Your Artificial Sweetner," in the 12/18/02 issue of *Don't Waste Arizona, Inc.*, Mary Nash Stoddard, Food Safety Expert and Author states, "Aspartame may be the unidentified environmental trigger for: Brain Tumors – Chronic Fatigue Syndrome – Lyme Disease, PMS – Migraine – Mild to Severe Depression – Carpal Tunnel – Arthritis – Meniere's – MS (Multiple Schlerosis) – Epilepsy – Anxiety/Phobia Disorders – Alzheimer's – ALS (Lou Gehrig's Disease) – Eosinophilia Myalgia Syndrome (EMS) – Graves Disease – Tinnitus – Fibromyalgia – Stroke – Heart Disease – Lupus – Mental Illness – Attention Deficit Disorder – other "Difficult-to-Diagnose Diseases." The article goes on to state that Asparatic Acid, which is 40 percent of the molecule in aspartame can change DNA and cause holes in the brains of lab animals. The article also states that aspartame can be especially hazardous to anyone with a preexisting medical condition such as diabetes.

Read your labels. There is a multitude of products on the market that contain aspartame.

Salt – How the Facts Shake Out

There are many people who feel they must salt their food. There are those who don't even taste their food before salting it! While they are under the impression that they are enhancing the taste of the food, they are actually masking the flavor. (Cigarettes also inhibit your taste buds).

When I eliminated salt from my diet, a whole new world of flavors opened up to me. My taste buds have become very sensitive. For one thing, many processed foods such as bread taste very salty to me. Many foods are so lacking in taste after processing that salt and sugar are added in large quantities. Many processed foods that you wouldn't even expect have large quantities of salt, sugar or both. As always, be sure to read the labels on the products you buy. I have found the same problem with some restaurant food. There have been times that the taste is so salty it is not enjoyable. I now order items to specifically avoid salt. Most restaurants are very accommodating.

Interesting Note

There's a question up for debate as to whether processed foods should even be allowed to be called foods. That includes so-called "enriched" foods. During refining and processing, they are pumped full of sugar, salt, artificial flavorings and colorings, additives, preservatives and hydrogenated or partially hydrogenated oil. Did I leave anything out? Oh yes... They are acid and mucus producing foods which contain no fiber!

Make it your goal to eliminate added salt to any foods. Aside from the health hazards, including hardening of the cells of tissues and organs which contributes to high blood pressure, those of you who are interested in maintaining a smooth, wrinkle-free skin might want to take note here. Excess salt contributes to dry, wrinkled skin.

Consuming excess salt leads to thirst and more water consumption, resulting in bloating. This water retention then inhibits the elimination of toxic salts from the body. This excess fluid can lead to inflammation of the connective tissues in the joints, which inhibits motion and causes pain similar to that of arthritis.

Salt is one of the greatest robbers of calcium in our bodies. This is a serious concern, especially to women at high risk of osteoporosis (such as those going through menopause) and bone fractures.

Health Hint

Just the burger patty from a fast food restaurant contains approximately 1,200 mg of sodium!

According to Jean Carper in her book *Food – Your Miracle Medicine,* "Sodium has long been hailed to be a cancer threat to the stomach, especially when combined with other carcinogens, such as residues and smoke from barbecuing and grilling meat. Cured meats, such as hot dogs, ham, cold cuts and bacon are also high in sodium. Salt appears particularly virulent when the diet is also low in fruits and vegetables that may counteract the cancer process."

It has been reported that approximately 75% of the sodium in the food supply is found in processed foods. It is present in almost every canned and frozen item, cake, cookie, sauce, bread and dairy product that you buy. You might even be surprised to find that it is even found in candy. Always read labels when shopping!

There is enough naturally occurring sodium in the raw living plant foods I eat that I don't need to add any sodium to my diet. A list of these foods is included in the Minerals section of the Appendix.

Health Hint

Enhance the natural salt in foods by using garlic, herbs, spices and lemon. If you must use salt, try to use Celtic sea salt. It is minimally processed and will draw out and intensify the flavors in your cooking. Common table salt is highly processed and contains additives to keep it free-flowing.

Caffeine

We have a love affair with our coffees. Not just the strong and dark variety, but with specialty coffees galore. There are cappuccinos, lattes, and all sorts of flavored coffees. The list goes on and on. We take a "coffee break" to relax. If we don't drink coffee, we may drink tea or cola. The trouble is, caffeine doesn't relax us, it stimulates us and is addicting.

There are a host of other negative effects caffeine may be responsible for in our bodies. Because caffeine is a diuretic, it causes us to lose fluids from our bodies. It is dehydrating and important minerals are lost through this process.

Women may experience fibrocystic breasts and uterine fibroids. Our nervous systems are negatively affected and we may experience anxiety, insomnia and/or hyperactivity.

For those of you who love your coffee, tea or cola, weaning off from these products may be a little rough. For the coffee and tea bunch, try mixing your regular drink with a decaffeinated drink. Keep increasing the amount of decaffeinated drink until the caffeine is eliminated.

I don't really recommend drinking decaffeinated coffee because it has been processed with chemical substances. Even when the package states "naturally decaffeinated," there is no guarantee. However, if someone is going to drink decaffeinated coffee, I would recommend that they buy coffee that has been decaffeinated though the "Swiss Water Process" method. This patented method does not use chemicals.

PART 4

Recipes
and
Menus

RECIPES "ON THE GO"

I prefer to keep my meals very simple to maximize nutrient absorption. I rarely fix recipes unless entertaining. The following are just a few simple recipes you might enjoy. There are many publications out on vegetarian recipes, if you would like to pursue this further.

Beverages

Cantaloupe Shake

This is one of my all-time favorites. I take the ripe inside fruit from the entire cantaloupe, dice it, and put it in a blender with about 1/4 cup cold water. Blend it on high speed for about a minute and you have a very delicious drink. You won't want to go back to a regular milk shake after this.

Cantaloupe is a cleansing fruit with a very high water content. I promise you this is good. I haven't found anyone yet who has not liked this one.

Apple/Orange/Banana Shake

Take an apple, a peeled orange and a peeled banana, dice them and put them in a blender. Blend until smooth. Believe it or not, the combination is great!

Apples are high in fiber and help lower cholesterol. Oranges are a natural cancer inhibitor and are also rich in antioxidant vitamin C and Beta-carotene. Bananas soothe the stomach and have an antibiotic effect.

I realize it flies in the face of my advice of not mixing acid (citrus) and sweet (banana) fruits together, but I have never had a problem with this drink. Neither has anyone else that I have served this to. It is an energy packed starter for the day.

Watermelon Shake

I prepare this the same way I prepare the cantaloupe shake. You may not need to add additional water. Watermelon is cleansing, and contains lycopene and glutathione, antioxidant and anti-cancer compounds. It is also mildly anti-bacterial.

Make Up Your Own Shake

I am constantly experimenting. Try any combination of berries, or fruits. You may want to add a little water. You never know what you will come up with but, I can assure you, you can almost never go wrong. Remember the more vibrant the color, the more nutrients and antioxidants contained in the fruit

A Note About Green Tea

New research shows that the antioxidants in green tea may reduce the risk of heart disease and certain cancers. This does not apply to herbal teas. However, they are a still a good source of water.

Simple Meals

Veggies in a Pita

INGREDIENTS:
- 2 whole wheat pitas
- 1/2 cup of veggie refried beans
- 1/3 cup salt-free salsa
- 2 each red and yellow pepper, chopped
- 1 large sweet onion, chopped
- Large olives, sliced
- 2 small tomatoes, chopped
- 1/4 avocado, chopped
- Cold pressed extra virgin olive oil
- 1 teaspoon Cilantro, chopped

DIRECTIONS:
Cut the pitas open halfway. Mix refried beans and salsa and spread on the pitas. Mix chopped onion, peppers, tomatoes and cilantro. Fill pitas with mixture and add chopped olives. Drizzle with olive oil. If you like sour cream, you may want to try a soy-based sour cream.
Serves 2

Avocado Lover's Sandwich

I eat a lot of avocados. They are easy to digest, the fat is monounsaturated, contains antioxidants, and are rich in potassium and wonderful for the skin.

INGREDIENTS:
- 2 slices sprouted grain bread
- 1 avocado, sliced and peeled
- 2 teaspoons vegan mayonnaise* or flax seed oil
- 1/4 cup bean sprouts
- 2 slices tomato
- 1 slice firm tofu or non-dairy cheese
- 4 teaspoons sunflower seeds (optional)

DIRECTIONS:
Spread mayonnaise or drizzle flax seed oil on the bread. Sprinkle the sunflower seeds on. Add Tofu or non-dairy cheese, tomato, avocado and sprouts.
Serves 1.

*You can find vegan mayonnaise in most health food stores

Yummy Hummus

INGREDIENTS:
- 1 1/3 cup dried chickpeas
- 1/2 cup fresh lemon juice (or add to taste)
- 3 tablespoons cold pressed extra-virgin olive oil
- 1/2 teaspoon salt
- 4 cloves garlic, pressed or crushed
- 1/4 teaspoon ground cumin
- 1/2 cup Tahini (sesame seed paste)

DIRECTIONS:
Rinse chickpeas and drain. Place in pan or bowl and cover with water. Let stand for 5 hours to overnight. Drain chickpeas and add clean water to about an inch above the chickpeas. Bring to boil. Reduce heat to low and simmer uncovered until the chickpeas become very tender and the skins begin to crack (approximately 60 minutes). Remove from heat and drain. Save the liquid from cooking.

Using a blender or food processor, combine all the ingredients and blend until the mixture is soft and creamy. You can add a bit of the cooking liquid to make the mixture creamier if necessary. Add more lemon to taste.

Serves 6-8.

Yummy Hummus Sandwich

INGREDIENTS:
- 2 slices sprouted grain bread
- Hummus
- Tomatoes, sliced
- Cucumber, sliced
- Mushroom, sliced
- Avocado, sliced
- Sprouts
- Red onion, sliced (optional)

DIRECTIONS:
Spread layer of hummus on both slices of bread. Layer the veggies. Put together and enjoy!

Serves 1.

Greek Lettuce Wraps

INGREDIENTS:
- Tomatoes, diced
- Cucumbers, diced
- Onion, diced
- Cold pressed extra virgin olive oil
- Fresh lemon juice
- Fresh basil
- Olives
- Firm tofu, diced into small cubes
- Lettuce leaves, washed (try to use the dark green variety – more nutrients)

DIRECTIONS:
Mix veggies, basil, olives, oil and lemon juice. Spoon into the lettuce leaves. Add a few olives and cubes of tofu. Roll cabbage roll style.

Garden Gazpacho

This cold soup originated in Spain. There are many varia-tions on this soup. It is spicy, tasty and a powerhouse of nutri-tion. Add other vegetables if you desire. Make your own varia-tion!

INGREDIENTS:
- 4 cups ripe tomatoes, diced
- 1-2 large, ripe avocados, peeled and sliced
- 1 each medium red, yellow and green pepper, seeded and diced
- 2 cucumbers, peeled and diced
- Juice of 1 lemon (the juice of a fresh lime will also work)
- 3-4 stalks celery, diced
- 2-3 tablespoons cold pressed virgin olive oil
- 1/4 cup parsley, chopped
- 1/4 cup cilantro or basil, chopped
- 1 pinch Celtic sea salt
- 1 pinch pepper
- Several drops Tabasco sauce (optional)
- 2-3 cups purified cold water (vary to taste)

DIRECTIONS:

Put all ingredients *except the avocados* in a blender. Process until well blended. Season to taste and serve chilled. Garnish the soup with avocado slices (This is not only decorative but also adds staying power, essential fatty acids and additional nu-trients).
Serves 4-6

Fresh Onion Soup

INGREDIENTS:
- 1 onion or bunch scallions, chopped
- 1 tablespoon cold pressed extra virgin olive oil
- 6-8 cups fresh greens, chopped
  (spinach, chard, Chinese cabbage, bok choy, etc.)
- 4 cups vegetable broth
- Salt and pepper

DIRECTIONS:

Lightly sauté onion in oil until very soft. Add broth and greens. Simmer until they wilt. Add salt and pepper to taste.

This is a very basic soup recipe. You can add variety to this soup by adding one or more of your favorite vegetables *before* simmering the greens. Add the greens *after* the other vegetables are soft. Try some of the following:

- Carrots, lightly steamed
- Celery, chopped or sliced
- Potatoes, cubed & lightly steamed
- Yellow squash, diced
- Zucchini, sliced

TRANSITION MENUS

Everyone must walk this path at his or her own rate. Some will be ready to make great leaps, others will want to take small steps. But, if followed diligently, all who walk this path, regardless of which transition level they choose, will ultimately succeed and benefit in every area of their lives.

The following are *sample menus*. You may substitute or eliminate foods as long as you keep the general basis of the meal the same. For example, if you would like to substitute apple juice for grapefruit juice, go ahead. If you would like to substitute Brazil nuts for pumpkin seeds, that's fine too. You get the idea. These are sample menus and the elements of proper food combining have not been strictly adhered to.

It should be noted that processed foods, hydrogenated fats and oils, refined sugar and salt should not be included or used as a substitute. Try to keep any beverage with a meal to a very small amount of water. Buy organic meats and vegetables whenever possible. If organic products are not available, wash thoroughly before eating.

Salad Dressing Tips

• Squeeze a fresh orange over your salad. The combination of the dark leafy greens and the orange tastes great and you are getting antioxidant power and vitamin C! The orange juice also stimulates the production of natural hydrochloric acid in the stomach which aids in the digestion of the greens.

• Use olive oil or flax oil with fresh lemon juice for a dressing. Neither of these contain additives, preservatives, chemicals, processed sugar or salt.

Transition 1 Menus

This menu is for the person who chooses to continue to eat meat and dairy products while cutting down on the portions. The remainder of the diet would include fruits, vegetables, nuts, seeds, whole grains, and legumes.

Monday

Breakfast:	Fresh Fruit Juice
	Eggs (preferably boiled)
	Cooked Oatmeal with Dried Fruit
Lunch:	Pineapple Rings and Cottage Cheese
Dinner:	Fresh Fruit Juice (consumed 15 minutes before the meal)
	Large Green Salad with Several Types of Raw Vegetables
	Small Baked Potato
	Chicken Breast

Tuesday

Breakfast	Chamomile Tea
	Fresh Fruit Juice
	Slice of Sprouted Grain Toast with Mashed Avocado
Lunch:	Omelet Filled with Lightly Steamed Vegetables
Dinner:	Large Green Salad with Several Types of Raw Vegetables
	Small Salmon Steak
	Lightly Steamed Green Beans
	Slice of Sourdough Bread

Wednesday

Breakfast: Fresh Fruit Juice
Herbal Tea
Fruit-Sweetened Granola with Rice Milk

Lunch: Whole Grain Pancakes with Maple Syrup
Apple
Low-Fat Cottage Cheese

Dinner: Fresh Fruit Juice (consume 15 minutes before eating meal)
Large Green Salad with Several Types of Raw Vegetables
Veggie Burger (Soy Based) with Lettuce, Tomato and Onion, on a Slice of Sourdough Bread

Thursday

Breakfast: Fresh Fruit Juice
Yogurt with Fresh Strawberries
Herbal Tea
Slice Melon

Lunch: Unsalted Rye-Crisp with Low Fat or Soy or Nut Cheese Slices
Sliced Banana with Rice Milk
Celery and Carrot Sticks.

Dinner: Large Green Salad with Several Types of Raw Vegetables
Fresh Onion Soup with Sourdough Bread Slices
Baked Banana Squash

Friday

Breakfast: Banana and Orange Slices
Slice Sprouted Grain Toast with Nut Butter
Herb Tea of Your Choice

Lunch: Fruit Smoothie
Turkey Slice on Sprouted Grain Bread
Carrot and Cucumber Slices

Dinner: Large Green Salad with Several Types of Raw Vegetables
Small Grilled Fresh Tuna Steak
Baked Potato

Transition 2 Menus

Meat, as well as processed foods, preservatives, chemicals, hydrogenated fats, sugar and salt have been eliminated from this person's diet. The dairy consumption is minimal. This person is naturally eating smaller portions and less food overall.

Monday

Breakfast: Fresh Fruit Juice
             Strawberries and Bananas
Lunch: Fresh Vegetable Juice
             Hummus and Diced Tomatoes and Cucumber
               in Organic Whole Grain Pita
Dinner: Fresh Fruit Juice (consume 15 minutes before
               eating meal)
             Steamed Vegetables of Choice
             Brown Rice
             Leafy Green Salad

Tuesday

Breakfast: Fruit Smoothie (Banana, Apple and Orange)
             Yogurt with Strawberries
Lunch: Herbal Tea
             Sliced Tomatoes and Slices of Low Fat Mozza-
               rella Cheese Drizzled with Olive Oil
             Steamed Broccoli
Dinner: Fresh Vegetable Juice
             Large Green Salad with Several Types of Raw
               Vegetables
             Carrot and Celery Sticks
             Fresh Vegetable Soup
             Sourdough Bread Slice

Wednesday

Breakfast: Fresh Fruit Juice
             Soy Yogurt with Banana Slices
             Slice of Sprouted Grain Sesame Seed Bread

Lunch:	Herbal Tea
	Cottage Cheese with Fresh Pineapple and Strawberries
	Baked Crackers
Dinner:	Fresh Vegetable Juice
	Lightly Sautéed Vegetables and Extra Firm Tofu
	Brown Rice
	Leafy Green Salad

Thursday

Breakfast:	Melon Slice
	Fresh Fruit Juice
	Celery Sticks Filled with Nut Butter
Lunch:	Mashed Avocado
	Salt-Free Fresh Salsa
	Baked Corn Chips
Dinner:	Lettuce Wraps Filled with Chopped, Sautéed Vegetables and Drizzled with Fresh Lemon and Olive Oil
	Baked Crackers
	Baked Banana Squash

Friday

Breakfast:	Oatmeal with Rice Milk and Berries
	Fresh Fruit Juice
	Sliced Peach
Lunch:	Herbal Tea
	Baked Yam
	Steamed Asparagus
	Slice of Tempeh
Dinner:	Fresh Vegetable Juice
	Soy Burger with Whole Grain Bun and Fresh Burger Toppings

Transition 3 Menus

This diet is mostly raw plant-based foods (full of the life-force). The juices are made from fresh fruits and vegetables. No meat, dairy products, processed foods, chemicals, preservatives, additives, sugar, salt or grains are consumed. Fresh vegetables, fruits, nuts, seeds, soy products and pure water are consumed. This way of eating will provide you with incredible health and beauty benefits. The only step higher than this would be a 100% raw plant-based diet. Many people will choose to remain at this level. You will find that your body requires less food and simple meals.

Important Note:

This is only a sample menu. Some people will require more concentrated foods such as an avocado in the mornings to keep their blood sugar level consistent and avoid energy dips. Others will do fine and feel the lightest and most energetic by starting their day with fruits only. Some might choose to start their day with a salad. You will find what works best for you by using your Food Journal as a guide and trying different combinations. I will occasionally have cooked squash or baked potatoes. I find that my body will have a craving for something warm, especially in the winter. When it does, I listen and provide my body with what it is asking for. The point here is to provide maximum health for our bodies, not to become slaves to rigid rules.

Monday

Breakfast: Fresh Juice Made from an Orange/Apple/Banana
                       Sunflower Seeds

Lunch: Apple
                       Celery Sticks with Nut Butter
                       Herb Tea

Dinner: Large Green Salad with Several Raw Vegetables
                       Topped with Cubed Tofu and Avocado Slices

Tuesday

Breakfast: Melon
                       Fresh Juice

Lunch:	Green Salad Topped with Alfalfa Sprouts and Pumpkin Seeds
Dinner:	Fresh Fruit Juice
	Fresh Vegetable Platter Drizzled with Sesame Oil
	Herb Tea

Wednesday

Breakfast:	Fresh Apple Juice
	Grapes
	Celery with Nut Butter
Lunch:	Garden Gazpacho (Cold Spanish Vegetable Soup)
	Walnuts
	Plum
Dinner:	Baked Banana Squash
	Tomato/Cucumber/Celery Salad

Thursday

Breakfast:	Fresh Grapefruit Juice
	Banana Slices
Lunch:	Avocado and Tomato Slices Drizzled with Olive Oil
	Celery with Nut Butter
Dinner:	Large Spinach Salad Topped with Sesame Seeds, Drizzled with Sesame Oil and a Touch of Light Rice Vinegar
	Tempeh Slices

Friday

Breakfast:	Berry/Banana Smoothie
	Mango Slices
	Raw Cashews
Lunch:	Raw Vegetable Plate Drizzled with Olive Oil, Sprinkled with Sliced Almonds
Dinner:	Fresh Lettuce Wraps Filled with Several Types of Chopped Vegetables and Mashed Avocado, Drizzled with Olive Oil
	Herb Tea of Choice
	Olives

CONCLUSION:

It's All About Choice – *Yours*

*"Choose to live your life as an inspiration to oth-
ers... when you are your best, you are the most positive model for others to emulate. Your life is a re-
flection about how you feel about and treat yourself. Be true to yourself."*
– Author Unknown

We've traveled this journey together so far. It is now time for
you to sprout your own wings. But remember: you are never
alone. You exist in a loving, giving universe that is waiting to
fulfill your desires. Remember also that even though it is loving
and giving, it responds to your choices whether they are empowering or defeating. I have become absolutely aware of the
truth of this in my own life. Keep your mind focused on what
you *want*, not what you *don't want*.

You now have all the tools you need to begin to live a life of
limitless fulfillment. There are two other basics that, if not mentioned, would make your information here incomplete. Those
two tools are belief and action. Information of any kind is only
of use when it is put into action. And to be put into action, one
must believe that he or she is capable of accomplishing the goal.

Be kind to yourself. Realize that you have made a life altering choice for the better. Changes will not happen overnight. But
when they begin happening, you will be almost overwhelmed
(pleasantly) with the positive things that begin happening in your
life. Along with shedding pounds and becoming more connected
with yourself, coincidences, chance happenings, intuitive guidance and happy surprises of all kinds begin to appear in your
life. You develop a solid feeling of self-trust which aids tremen-
dously in decision making because you know you are being
guided and watched over by a force much greater than you. It is
a wonderful feeling and one which eluded me all the years of my
life until I made the changes we have shared in this book.

Start with a diet that is 60% raw plant-based foods and 40%
cooked foods if that is what feels right. Move on to a 70%/30%
ratio and so on as your body tells you it is ready. Give yourself
4-6 weeks of loving attention and see the miraculous changes
that will begin to occur in your life. But, again, remember that

information is only important if it is used. It is so very important that I feel I must emphasize again that any information that just sits is virtually useless. It is when that information is combined with action and intention that profound results can and do occur. Amazing accomplishments are lying in wait inside each and every one of us, just waiting to unfold.

The necessary key is for each of us to accept that we have this power within ourselves. It is innate. We do not need to look outside to external sources to tell us what is right or to define who we are. The blueprint for a successful life is imprinted within each of us. Our mind, body and spirit will joyfully respond for our highest good when we listen to the voice within and use the *one great tool* we have each been given to use, no matter what our circumstances at the moment. That one great tool is *choice*. Choice in how you respond to situations, choice in what you believe, choice in who you associate with, choice in what you are willing to accept, choice in the amount of effort you are willing to expend to make things better, choice in looking on the bright or the dismal side of a situation. As you can see, *everything hinges on choice*. And choice is totally, 100% within your control. Choose right this very minute to be open to change and growth and to let the best in you unfold. Magical leaps and bounds will start occurring in your self-respect and all other areas of your life.

My great desire in writing this book is to pass on to you what I have discovered for myself in hopes that it will bring you the joy and fulfillment it has brought — and continues to bring me — in an ever increasing way. It would have made such a difference for me if there had been someone who could have explained this program and given me some direction when I was making my lifestyle and attitude changes. It is my desire to be as much of a mentor to you as possible, covering the questions and issues that I faced. If you make the choice now to apply the principles of this book in your life, I promise that you will clearly understand why I have chosen to call this program *The Greatest Diet on Earth.*

APPENDIX:

Tables and References

The following section contains complete reference tables of the different foods discussed in this book. Refer to this information when creating your meals with raw plant-based foods.

ALKALINE FORMING FOODS

Alfalfa	Dates	Parsnips
Almonds	Eggplant	Peach
Apple	Figs	Pear
Apple Cider Vinegar	Flax Seeds	Peas
Apricot	Fruit Juices	Peppers
Asparagus	Garlic	Pineapple
Avocado	Grapefruit	Pumpkin
Bananas	Grapes	Pumpkin Seeds
Barley Grass	Green Tea	Rutabaga
Bee Pollen	Herbal Tea	Sea Veggies
Beets	Honeydew Melon	Spirulina
Berries (all kinds)	Kale	Sprouted seeds
Broccoli	Kohlrabi	Sprouts
Brussel Sprouts	Lemon	Squashes
Cabbage	Lettuce	Sunflower Seeds
Cantaloupe	Limes	Tangerines
Carrots	Mangos	Tempeh (fermented)
Cauliflower	Millet	Tofu (fermented)
Celery	Mineral Water	Tomatoes
Chard	Mushrooms	Vegetable Juices
Cherries	Mustard Greens	Water
Chestnuts	Nectarine	Watercress
Collard Greens	Onions	Wheat Grass
Cucumber	Orange	Wild Greens
Currants	Papayas	

ACID FORMING FOODS

Amaranth
Aspartame
Avocado Oil
Barley
Beef
Beer
Black Beans
Brazil Nuts
Canola Oil
Cashews
Chick Peas
Clams
Corn Oil

Cranberries
Fats & Oils
Fish
Flax Oil
Green Peas
Hard Liquor
Hemp Seed Oil
Kidney Beans
Lamb
Lard
Lentils
Lima Beans
Lobster

Nuts & Nut Butters
Olive Oil
Peanut Butter
Peanuts
Pecans
Pinto Beans
Rice Cakes
Safflower Oil
Tahini
Walnuts
Wine

NOTE: Drugs, chemicals and pesticides are also acid forming.

WATER CONTENT OF FOODS

Food	Water Content	Food	Water Content
Fruit:		*Vegetables:*	
Apricots	85%	Carrots	88%
Bananas	76%	Fresh Tomatoes	93%
Papayas	89%	Broccoli	91%
Peaches	90%	Parsley	86%
Pineapples	85%	Green Peppers	94%
Grapefruit	88%	Cauliflower	91%
Sweet Potatoes	71%	Egg Plant	92%
Watermelon	93%	Endive	94%
Cucumbers	96%	Lettuce	94%
Honeydew Melon	94%	Asparagus	93%
Tomatoes	94%	Celery	93%
Watermelons	94%	Watercress	91%
Bell Peppers	93%	Green Cabbage	90%
Cantaloupe	93%	Bok Choy	87%
Grapefruits	91%	Onion Root	87%
Okra	90%	Parsley	79%
Strawberries	89%	Kale	65%
Apricots	87%	Garlic Root	64%
Tangerines	87%		
Lemons	85%	*Nuts & Seeds (unsoaked):*	
Mulberries	85%	Almonds	7%
Apples	84%	Coconut water	92%
Oranges	84%	Coconut (young)	64%
Plums	84%	Coconut (mature)	35%
Mangos	83%	Almonds	26%
Pears	83%	Walnuts	25%
Raspberries	83%	Macadamias	18%
Blackberries	82%	Brazil Nuts	15%
Cherries	82%	Pine Nuts	15%
Lychees	82%	Sunflower Seeds	15%
Nectarines	80%		
Persimmons (soft)	80%		
Figs	79%		
Grapes	79%		
Prickly Pear	79%		
Huckleberries	78%		
Avocados	75%		
Olives(sun-ripened)	70%		
Dates(fresh)	55%		
Prunes (dried)	35%		

ALKALIZING FOODS AND THEIR CALCIUM CONTENT

Legumes:

Red bean, dried 110mg
Mung sprouts 118mg
Chickpea 150mg
Soybean, dried 226mg
Pea, green fresh 26mg
Soybean sprouts 48mg
Lima bean, fresh 52mg
Soybean, fresh 67mg
Lentil, dried 79mg

Nuts and Seeds (more acidic):

Sesame seed 1160mg
Almond 234mg
Filbert 209mg
Brazil nut 186mg
Sunflower seed 120mg
Pumpkin seed 51mg

Grains (more acidic):

Wheat bran 119mg
Wheat 46mg
Barley 34mg
Rice, brown 32mg
Millet 20mg

Fruits:

Grapefruit 16mg
Tomato 13mg
Avocado 10mg
Lemon juice 7mg

Vegetables:

Seaweed, agar 567mg
Seaweed, dulse 296mg
Collards(leaves) 250mg
Kale(leaves) 249mg
Turnip greens 246mg
Parsley 203mg
Mustard greens 183mg
Watercress 151mg
Beet greens 119mg
Broccoli 103mg
Fennel 100mg
Rhubarb 96mg
Spinach 93mg
Okra 92mg
Chard, Swiss 88mg
Cress 81mg
Lettuce, loose-leaf 68mg
Leek 52mg
Artichoke 51mg
Onion(green) 51mg
Cabbage 43mg
Celery 39mg
Brussels sprouts 36mg
Lettuce, Boston 35mg
Radish 30mg
Garlic 29mg
Cauliflower 25mg
Cucumber 25mg
Asparagus 21mg
Lettuce, Iceberg 20mg
Bamboo shoots 13mg
Pepper, red 13mg
Eggplant 12mg
Pepper, green 9mg

VITAMINS

The following are vitamins you should be familiar with. This information will give you a brief overview of their beneficial effects on the body and some good food sources.

Vitamin A

Benefits:

Beta-carotene (natural orange pigment) is an antioxidant that is converted to Vitamin A by the body and is produced by plants. It fights the free radicals in your body. Vitamin A is necessary for healthy eyes, teeth, hair and smooth, disease-free skin. It is very important for the health of the immune system. It helps prevent infections by boosting the infection fighting actions of the white blood cells.

Food Sources:

Apricots
Avocado
Broccoli
Brussels sprouts
Butternut Squash
Cantaloupe
Carrots*
Collards
Endive
Hubbard squash
Kale
Mangos
Mustard greens
Napa Cabbage
Nectarines
Pumpkin

Romaine lettuce
Savoy cabbage
Spinach
Sweet Potatoes
Swiss chard
Tangerines
Tomatoes
Turnip Greens
Watermelon

*One carrot per day has double your RDA

B Complex

Benefits:
Very important to the nervous and digestive systems and to the enzyme process in the body. Reduces facial oiliness, the formation of blackheads and helps keep the skin vibrant. Vitamin B Folacin plays a key role in the formation of red blood cells. The body is rather easily depleted of this complex by stress and can be easily lost in food by cooking and processing. Coffee, alcohol and tea can wash this vitamin from the body.

Food Sources:
Acorn squash
Asparagus
Avocado
Bananas
Broccoli
Brussels sprouts
Butternut squash
Cauliflower
Dark leafy greens
Fish
Honeydew
Mangos
Potatoes
Raisins
Spinach
Sunflower seeds
Sweet potatoes
Watermelon*
Whole Grains

*High in beta carotene

Vitamin C

Benefits:
Acts as an antioxidant. Necessary for collagen production, healing wounds, immune system.

Food Sources:

Acorn squash	Napa Cabbage
Apples	Nectarines
Apricots	Okra
Artichokes	Onions
Asparagus	Oranges
Avocado	Papayas
Beets	Parsley*
Blackberries	Parsnips
Blueberries	Pears
Broccoli	Peppers
Brussels sprouts	Pineapple
Butternut squash	Plums
Cabbage	Potatoes
Cantaloupe	Pumpkin
Cauliflower	Radishes
Celery	Raspberries
Collards	Red Cabbage
Cranberries	Romaine lettuce
Grapefruit	Rutabagas
Green peas	Savoy cabbage
Honeydew	Snap beans
Hubbard squash	Spinach
Kale	Strawberries**
Kiwi fruit	Sweet potatoes
Kohlrabi	Swiss chard
Leeks	Tomatoes
Lemons	Turnip greens
Limes	Turnips
Mangos	Watermelon
Mustard greens	

* Also provides B vitamin Folacin
** Collagen booster

Vitamin E

Benefits:
Act as an antioxidant. Supports cell membrane and cell tissues. Improves circulation in tiny face capillaries and is important in healing because it aids in the replacement of cells on the skin's surface. Important for healthy circulatory system. Boosts the immune system.

Food Sources:
Asparagus
Avocado
Dark leafy green vegetables
Grains
Nuts
Olives
Polyunsaturated plant oils
Seeds
Spinach
Sweet potatoes
Tofu
Wheat germ

Vitamin K

Benefits:
Regulates blood calcium and the synthesis of the blood-clotting proteins. Vitamin K is also made by bacteria that are always present in the intestinal tract.

Food Sources:
Cabbage
Cauliflower
Dark green leafy vegetables
Soybean.
Spinach

MINERALS

Minerals are critical to good health. They are essential to the normal functioning of vitamins and nutrients in the body.

Calcium

Benefits:
Necessary for formation of bones and teeth. Important in the fight against osteoporosis in menopausal women. Supports blood clotting. Menstrual cramp inhibitor.

Food Sources:

Broccoli	Sesame seeds
Carrots	Spinach
Figs	Tofu
Kale	
Parsley	
Sardines	

Chromium

Benefits:
Associated with insulin. It is important in the release of energy from glucose.

Food Sources:

Nuts	Whole grains
Polyunsaturated vegetable oils	

Copper

Benefits:
Necessary for absorption and utilization of iron. Supports hemoglobin and enzyme formation. Important in maintaining elasticity and firmness of skin.

Food Sources:

Mushrooms	Seafood
Soy products	Wheat germ

Iodine

Benefits:
Important in the healthy functioning of the thyroid gland. This affects the metabolic rate of the body.

Food Sources:
Brazil nuts
Cod
Kelp

Iron

Benefits:
An important component of hemoglobin (blood). Iron also resides in muscle tissue. Vitamin C improves the ability to absorb iron from plant sources. Very important if anemic or menstruating, however, supplementation can be dangerous otherwise. For example, post-menopausal women are not losing iron-rich blood every month so the supplemental iron could start building up in their bodies, possibly speeding up the aging process, adding to the chances of heart disease, etc.

Food Sources:
Avocados
Barley grass
Beans
Beets
Dark green, leafy vegetables
Dried apricots
Grapes
Kelp
Pumpkin seeds
Raisins
Seaweed
Spinach
Wheat germ
Whole grain bread

Magnesium

Benefits:
Important for forming bones and teeth, reducing the risk of heart disease. Complements calcium in bone building. Important in building tooth enamel. Very important for women suffering PMS or peri-menopausal symptoms.

Food Sources:

Almonds	Legumes
Avocado	Soy beans
Brown rice	Spinach
Corn	Sunflower seeds
Dark, leafy, green vegetables	Swiss chard
Evening primrose oil	Tofu
Halibut	Wheat germ
Hazelnuts	

Manganese

Benefits:
Important for healthy bones, joint health, sex hormone production and immune cells. This is a component of the antioxidant enzyme superoxide dismutase (S.O.D.).

Food Sources:
Avocados
Beets
Green vegetables
Nuts
Peas
Pineapple
Pumpkin seeds
Whole grains

Phosphorous

Benefits:
Important in healthy bone formation and in energy conversion reactions in the body. Helps calm nerves. Heightens mental process. Important for teeth, hair, skin and bones.

Food Sources:
Almonds
Peanuts
Pumpkin Seeds
Sardines
Sesame seeds
Soy beans
Wheat germ

Potassium

Benefits:
Important in maintaining electrolyte balance. Contributes to nerve impulse transmission and muscle contractions.

Food Sources:

Acorn squash	Dates	Pumpkin
Apricots	Eggplant	Raisin
Artichokes	Figs	Raspberries
Asparagus	Honeydew	Spinach
Avocado	Hubbard squash	Strawberries
Bananas	Kale	Sweet potatoes
Beets	Kiwi	Tomatoes
Brussels sprouts	Kohlrabi	Watermelon
Butternut squash	Mangos	
Cabbage	Nectarines	
Carrots	Oranges	
Cauliflower	Papaya	
Celery	Parsnips	
Collard greens	Pears	
Corn	Potatoes	
Cucumbers	Prunes	

Selenium

Benefits:
Helps protect cell tissues and membranes. Important for healthy liver and heart function. It is also an important constituent of the antioxidant enzyme glutathione peroxidase. Works with Vitamin E.

Food Sources:
Brazil nuts (very good source)
Fish
Garlic
Nuts
Rice
Shellfish
Vegetables
Whole grains

Silicon (Silica)

Benefits:
Maintains integrity of blood vessel walls, cartilage, connective tissue and formation of healthy bones. Important in structure of hair and nails. Important in maintaining skin elasticity because it is involved in collagen production.

Food Sources:
Alfalfa sprouts
Bananas
Dark green vegetables
Onions
Root vegetables

Sodium

Benefits:
Important in muscle contraction and nerve impulse transmissions. Maintains fluid and electrolyte balance.

Food Sources:

Artichokes	Celery
Beets	Romaine lettuce
Broccoli	Snap beans
Cabbage	Spinach
Carrots	Sweet potatoes
Cauliflower	Turnips

Sulfur

Benefits:
Important in formation of hair, joints and nails. It is in the structure of most proteins and enzymes. Works with Vitamin B-complex in building tissue.

Food Sources:

Asparagus	Kidney beans
Broccoli	Legumes
Brussels sprouts	Lentils
Cabbage	Onions
Dried peaches	Shellfish
Garlic	Sprouts
Green peppers	Wheat germ

Zinc

Benefits:
Important in a large number of enzyme reactions. Important in normal cell division and function. Helps retard aging since it is essential in the formation of collagen. Important for insulin release. Important for healthy ovaries and prostate function. Necessary for healthy vision, taste and smell. Also part of the formation of the antioxidant enzyme superoxide dismutase (S.O.D.).

Food Sources:
Broccoli
Fish
Lentils
Mung beans
Pumpkin seeds
Pumpkin seeds
Sesame seeds
Shellfish
Spinach
Spirulina
Sunflower seeds
Tofu
Wheat germ
Whole grain bread
Whole oatmeal

BIBLIOGRAPHIES

Yeager, Selene. *New Foods For Healing.*
Emmaus, Pennsylvania: Rodale Press, Inc., 1998.

Jones, Susan Smith, Ph.D. *The Main Ingredients of Health & Happiness.*
Nevada City, CA: Dawn Publications, 1995.

Atkins, Robert C., M.D., *Dr. Atkins Age-Defying Diet Revolution.*
New York, NY: St. Martin's Press, 2000.

Stoppard, Miriam, Dr. *Natural Menopause.*
New York, NY: DK Publishing, 1998.

Null, Gary. *The Food-Mood-Body Connection.*
New York, NY: Seven Stories Press, 2000.

Stein, Diane. *The Natural Remedy Book for Women.*
Freedom, CA: The Crossing Press, 1992.

Prevention Magazine Health Books. *Age Erasers for Women.*
Emmasu, PA: Rodale Press, 1994.

Berkson, D. Lindsey. *Natural Answers for Women's Health Questions.*
New York, NY: Simon & Schuster, 2002.

Somer, Elizabeth, M.A., R.D. *The Origin Diet.*
New York, NY: Henry Holt & Co., 2001.

Null, Gary, Ph.D. *Ultimate Lifetime Diet.*
New York, NY: Broadway Books, 2000.

Gault-McNemee, Dorothy, M.D. *God's Diet.*
New York, NY: Random House, Inc., 1999.

Young, Robert & Young, Shelley Redford. *The ph Miracle.*
New York, NY: Warner Books, 2002.

Mindell, Earl, R.Ph., Ph.D. *Earl Mindell's Food As Medicine.*
New York, NY: Simon & Schuster, 1994.

Carper, Jean, *Food – Your Miracle Medicine.*
New York, NY: HarperCollins, 1993.

Null, Gary, Ph.D. *Ultimate Anti-Aging Program.*
New York, NY: Kensington Publishing Corp., 1999.

Haas, Elson, M.D., *The Detox Diet.*
Berkeley, CA: Celestial Arts, 1996

Wolfe, David, *Eating For Beauty.*
San Diego, CA: Maul Brothers Publishing, 2002

Anderson, Nina and Peiper, Howard, *Over 50, Looking 30!*
East Canaan, CT: Safe Goods, 1996

Nison, Paul, *Raw Knowledge.*
Brooklyn, NY: 343 Publishing Company, 2002

Cousens, Gabriel, Dr., *Spiritual Nutrition And The Rainbow Diet.*
San Rafael, CA: Cassandra Press, 1986

Batmanghelidj, F., M.D., *Your Body's Many Cries For Water.*
Falls Church, VA: Global Health Solutions, 1997

Joseph, James A., Ph.D., and Nadeau, Daniel, A., M.D., and
Underwood, Anne, *The Color Code.* New York, NY: Hyperion, 2002

Gittleman, Ann Louise, M.S., C.N.S., *The Living Beauty Detox Program.*
New York, NY: Harper Collins Publishing, 2000

Bonsteel, Alan, M.D., *Stay Young, Start Now.*
Berkeley, CA: Celestial Arts, 2000

Diamond, Marilyn and Schnell, Donald Burton, Dr., *Fitonics.*
New York, NY: Avon Books, 1996

Editors of Prevention Magazine, *Healing with Vitamins.*
Emmus, PA: Rodale Press, 1996

Roberts, Arthur M.D. and O'Brien, Mary E., M.D., *Nutraceuticals.*
New York, NY: The Berkeley Publishing Company, 2001

Wolfe, David, *The Sunfood Diet Success System.*
San Diego, CA: Maul Brothers Publishing, 2002

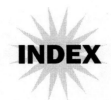

INDEX

S

T